CHRONIC PAIN, LOSS, AND SUFFERING

Loss and grief are an inherent part of chronic illness. But while much has been written on grief associated with death and dying, the grief and losses accompanying chronic illness have received relatively little scholarly attention. In this book, Ranjan Roy, a leading expert on chronic pain, addresses the complex issues related to loss among those with chronic illness.

For many patients with chronic pain disorders, the course of their illness is unpredictable and varied. Many seeming losses are transient and can be redeemed over time, for instance, through retraining and physical therapy, but are still serious and pose a challenge to the conventional understanding of the grief process. Indeed, clinical understanding of grief is undergoing a revolution. From its Freudian roots, it is shifting to a more social-psychological perspective. The phase-task approach to grief has come under serious scrutiny, and this book demonstrates some of the problems inherent in that conceptualization in its application to the chronically ill. In *Chronic Pain, Loss, and Suffering*, Roy evaluates the current state of knowledge through an examination of contemporary literature and clinical application. He presents a series of comprehensive case studies, which together indicate that the key challenge for many patients is loss of self-esteem and control. The chapters deal with a range of losses such as job loss, declining ability to function, loss of family and sexual roles, old age and its related losses, and suicide. Through discussion of the struggles and successes that chronically ill patients encounter in their journey, this work will assist clinicians in helping patients come to terms with the difficulties they face and to establish a renewed sense of self.

RANJAN ROY is a professor in the Faculty of Social Work and the Department of Clinical Health Psychology at the University of Manitoba and a consultant (scientific) in the Department of Anaesthesia at St Boniface Hospital in Winnipeg.

RANJAN ROY

Chronic Pain, Loss, and Suffering

UNIVERSITY OF TORONTO PRESS
Toronto Buffalo London

© University of Toronto Incorporated 2004
Toronto Buffalo London
Printed in Canada

ISBN 0-8020-3597-3

Printed on acid-free paper

National Library of Canada Cataloguing in Publication

Roy, Ranjan
  Chronic pain, loss and suffering/Ranjan Roy.

  Includes bibliographical references and index.
  ISBN 0-8020-3597-3

  1. Sickness – Psychology.   2. Chronic diseases – Psychological
  aspects.   3. Chronic pain – Psychological aspects.   4. Grief.
  5. Loss (Psychology).   I. Title.

  R726.5.R69 2004   616'.001'9   C2004-901370-X

University of Toronto Press acknowledges the financial assistance to its
publishing program of the Canada Council for the Arts and the Ontario Arts
Council.

University of Toronto Press acknowledges the financial support for its
publishing activities of the Government of Canada through the Book
Publishing Industry Development Program (BPIDP).

For Julian

Contents

Foreword DENNIS TURK   ix

Preface   xv

1 Loss and Grief: An Overview   3

2 Loss, Sadness, and Depression: Many Faces of Abnormal Grief and Other Complications   21

3 Job Loss and Chronic Illness: A Situation of Double Jeopardy   43

4 Declining Health and Functioning: Redefining Identity   62

5 Family Roles: What Is Lost?   82

6 Chronic Illness and Sexual Roles   103

7 Old Age, Pain, and Loss   124

8 Chronic Illness and Suicide: The Ultimate Loss   142

9 Grief Therapy   165

10 Epilogue   186

viii   Contents

References   193

Index   211

Foreword

DENNIS TURK

Chronic pain is a prevalent and costly problem for the individual pain sufferer, his or her family, and for society in general. Estimates suggest that 25 to 30 per cent of the population suffer from some chronic pain condition. These figures may be expected to escalate as the population ages and experiences the accompanying pain conditions such as osteoarthritis, osteoporosis, and peripheral neuropathies. Estimates for direct health care expenditures, indemnity costs, lost time from work, and lost tax revenue in the United States range from $150 (U.S. Bureau of the Census, 1996) to $215 billion (National Research Council, 2001). Of course, these astronomical figures cannot do justice to the incalculable human suffering of those with chronic pain. There is no question that chronic pain greatly impairs quality of life, causing significant physical disability and considerable emotional distress.

Despite the advances in the neurobiology of pain and the advent of new medications and technically sophisticated interventions, there appears to be no cure for the diverse set of chronic pain conditions on the horizon. Moreover, even the most advanced pharmacological preparations available only appear to reduce by approximately 35 per cent (Turk, 2002); a substantial percentage of patients treated with these drugs do not even achieve this level of benefit. In short, chronic pain is a generic classification that comprises a large, disabling set of conditions, and no treatment is currently available that can consistently or permanently eliminate or significantly palliate that pain for millions of sufferers. The person with chronic pain experiences symptoms, at least to some extent or anticipates them, 24 hours a day, 365 days a year, indefinitely. Chronic pain is, indeed, a chronic state similar in many ways to diabetes. As with all chronic conditions, people with chronic pain must assume a great deal of responsibility for self-management of their conditions.

The traditional biomedical view of chronic pain considers pain as a symptom of some underlying physical pathology, often located in a specific body part (e.g., knee, shoulder, back). Extensive efforts are undertaken to identify the source of pain – the 'pain generator.' The quest then is to identify the generator and either eliminate it or, if this cannot be accomplished, use surgical, pharmacological, or physical means to cut or block the nociceptive signals from reaching the brain – where they are perceived as pain. In a sense, the view is that of the body as a machine, and a body in pain is the result of some broken or worn-out part that needs to be fixed or replaced.

The traditional biomedical model that I have caricatured while focusing on the physical perturbations tends to neglect the fact that the symptom – pain – is perceived and is being reported by a conscious individual, with a life history that preceded the onset of the pain, who lives in a social context. As a result, there are a myriad of factors involved in the deceptively simple report of the patient's pain. Moreover, when pain persists over extended periods of time the symptoms come to be influenced by a range of affective, cognitive, behavioural, and environmental factors. The pain sufferer interprets the noxious sensations, and this interpretation is based on prior learning history, sociocultural context, current circumstances, and the availability of coping resources, social as well as financial. Pain sufferers' interpretations of the meaning of pain ('Will I ever be able to function like I did before the pain began?' or 'Will the pain persist and lead me to become an invalid?'), beliefs ('Physicians should be able to find and treat the cause' or 'I'm letting my family down'), attitudes ('I should not have to live this way!')

will contribute to their mood (e.g., fear, despair, anger), and behaviour ('If I perform household chores it will make my pain worse and might even lead to increased injury, thus, I should cease the activity').

Attitudes, beliefs, behaviours, and emotions can affect physiological functioning. For example, thoughts can contribute to emotional arousal that may induce muscle tension and exacerbation of pain. Avoidance of activity due to the belief that it will lead to additional damage may lead to further physical deconditioning. Continual passivity will prevent disconfirmation of the belief that hurt will inevitably lead to harm and confirm pain sufferers' views of themselves as being incapacitated. Reliance solely on medication may diminish the likelihood of undertaking self-management efforts (e.g., physical exercise, problem solving) and foster dependence on others.

Patients' moods and behaviours will, in turn, influence the responses of significant others. Family members may assume responsibilities; health care providers may initiate new treatments based on observation of the patient. Not only do significant others have an effect on the pain sufferer, the pain sufferer, too, has an influence on the mood as well as the behaviour of significant others. For example, one study (Flor, Turk, and Scholtz, 1987) reported that female spouses of male chronic pain patients were more depressed than the patients. There is a dynamic synergy between people with chronic illnesses and their significant others. Yet, little attention is given to the significant others, as they are far removed from the body part where pain is localized.

Consider the case of a forty-year-old truck driver who develops back pain. He now presents himself to a health care provider with a six-year history of symptoms. This man had a thirty-four-year history that pre-existed the onset of his pain. As part of that history he learned about pain and how symptoms are treated by observation of other family members, how he was treated and himself treated previous symptoms, and how the media present symptoms and the treatment of symptoms – be stoic, tough it out, obtain sympathy, relinquish responsibilities, anticipate treatment and resolution of symptoms, and so forth, depending on the types of experiences and information to which he was exposed during the thirty-four years preceding the onset of his symptoms.

Since the symptoms began six years ago, the truck driver has attempted to make sense of his condition, has been exposed to numerous diagnostic tests, treatments, and a great deal of advice from his family, friends, and health care providers. At first, he may have been optimistic, believing that the symptoms would abate on their own, reducing activities would lead to resolution of the cause of the symptoms, and time off work would permit his back to improve. Over time, with the persistence of symptoms, fear may have arisen; despite treatments and withdrawal from activities, his pain persists. He avoids physical activity, as this magnifies his pain, and as he withdraws from the activity he may notice less pain. Consequently, he learns to perform less and as a result becomes even more physically deconditioned.

As the truck driver is exposed to more and more futile tests to identify the cause of the symptoms, and with the failure of treatments, he may worry about his future; health care providers offer less hope, and family members become frustrated and distressed about the persistence of the symptoms with no end in sight. The truck driver is no longer working and has lost contact with former co-workers. His self-identity – a competent, employed, provider for his family – is challenged and his self-esteem and self-worth are diminished. He becomes demoralized and depressed, as does his family.

As we can see in the case of the truck driver, the cascade of events that began with the onset of symptoms are filtered through his prior experiences and are influenced by the set of events that were initiated following the onset of symptoms. It is not just his back that is the problem but his entire life is affected on every level – interpersonal, familial, social, recreational, emotional, behavioural, as well as physical. His perception of himself as a vigorous person who accepted familial and other responsibilities has changed. He has lost his role-identity, his self-esteem, his sense of self, and there is no end in sight.

The plight of the chronic pain sufferer is one permeated by loss, and this sense of loss contributes to the suffering accompanying the pain. No longer is it just the pain that is the problem but the implications that pain has on the person's ability to function both physically and emotionally and the person's perception of self-worth. Once all appropriate efforts to eliminate the problem are made and rehabilitation has been completed, the central problem for someone with chronic pain is overcoming grief related to the perceived losses, and finding meaning and acceptance of the loss of body functioning. People with persistent pain have to learn how to restructure their lives and identities to accommodate any residual physical limitations.

Despite the description of the truck driver, the majority of people with chronic pain – even those with significant physical limitations – find ways to cope and adapt, often heroically. Unfortunately, we know little about how they accomplish this. The tendency is to emphasize those who are referred for counselling because they are having difficulty. This group may actually be a minority, a significant minority nonetheless. It is this latter group that is the target of the present text.

In this volume, Professor Roy describes the set of losses and associated grief that accompany chronic pain. He uses clinical cases to illustrate how declining functioning, loss, and grief contribute to the suffering of chronic pain patients. He describes how coming to terms with the grief associated with the perceived and actual losses can help patients overcome the sense of suffering. He shows how the chronic pain patient may move from patient status to one of a person with chronic pain and accompanying limitations. Yet, self-identity and self-esteem can be restored – people with chronic pain may be different than they were before the onset of their symptoms but they can still achieve fulfilling lives. This is the primary point made in this book. It has an optimistic tone and key message. Even though chronic conditions confront people with significant challenges, they may be able to overcome the limitations and perceived losses. Resolution and accommodation can be achieved not as an end but as a process. To paraphrase Reinhold Niebuhr's

Serenity Prayer, people with chronic pain (all people actually) need the serenity to accept the things that they cannot change, the courage to change the things they can, and the wisdom to know the difference between the two. Professor Roy provides numerous illustrations showing how people with chronic pain can learn to assimilate and accommodate the accompanying losses, restoring and altering their self-identity as necessitated by their physical state, and thereby transcend their suffering.

REFERENCES

Flor, H., Turk D., and Scholz, O. (1987). Impact of chronic pain on the spouse: Marital, emotional, and physical consequences. *Journal of Psychosomatic Research*, 31: 63–72.

National Research Council. (2001). Musculoskeletal disorders and the workplace. Washington, DC: National Academy Press.

Turk, D. (2002). Clinical effectiveness and cost-effectiveness of treatments for patients with chronic pain. *Clinical Journal of Pain*, 18: 355–65.

United States Bureau of the Census. (1996). *Statistical Abstract of the United States: 1996*. (116th ed.). Washington, DC: author.

Preface

Loss and grief are an inherent part of chronic illness. Yet much of the grief literature is concentrated on grief associated with death, an irretrievable loss. Unlike death, many losses associated with chronic illness can be retrieved or at least partly recovered. Inability to function in one kind of job may result in retraining for more suitable work. Some losses are indeed permanent. Patients go through complex forms of grieving with their partial or total loss of roles and functions. The literature on this topic is sparse. There is very little recognition of the differences and similarities between grief associated with death and grief associated with losses that emanate from chronic illness.

In this volume, an effort has been made to draw that distinction. The key challenge for patients is the assault on their identity. This assault follows an unknown and often unpredictable course. Many patients manage to cope and function at almost normal levels despite their medical conditions. Then deterioration in their medical condition forces unwanted changes in their role functions. Loss of job, inability to perform routine household chores, loss of libido, and loss of many other valued and necessary roles are at the root of the challenge to the patient's sense of self. Much of this book is a discussion of the trials and tribulations and hope that chronically ill patients encounter in their journey.

Clinical understanding of grief is undergoing a revolution. From its Freudian roots, it is shifting more and more to a social–psychological perspective. The phase-task orientation of grief has come under serious scrutiny, and this book demonstrates some of the problems inherent in that conceptualization in its application to the chronically ill. This book has attempted to combine the current state of knowledge through a survey of contemporary literature with clinical application. The latter was achieved by comprehensive case illustrations.

I would like to thank my friend Brian Minty of the University of Manchester, England, for his sustained help in bringing this project to fruition. Margaret Roy acted as my main critic and provided valuable suggestions. Without the support of my editor Virgil Duff of the University of Toronto Press, this project may have never been published. He has my deepest gratitude. Finally, this project was made possible by a generous grant from the Faculty of Social Work Endowment Fund, University of Manitoba.

CHRONIC PAIN, LOSS, AND SUFFERING

1

Loss and Grief: An Overview

John Bowlby's seminal work (1981a, 1981b) on attachment, separation, and loss, in particular his original conceptualization of loss as being rooted in the mother-child relationship, has found wide application. Concepts of attachment and loss are covered in topics as varied as relocation of the elderly in a rural area to the loss of a limb, to loss of health, or to loss of a spouse.

First, however, we shall review briefly the original conceptualization of loss and grief as propounded by John Bowlby, its principal protagonist. Bowlby's treatment of loss had a central source, namely, separation from or death of a loved person, be it a child or spouse. He brought together a number of theoretical views and developed a coherent theory of loss. The predictable response to loss is mourning. Bowlby drew a distinction between healthy and pathological mourning, and compared the responses to loss of young children with adults. He noted that, generally, in the studies dealing with adult responses to loss the loss was mainly the death of someone. Hence, he devoted the third volume of his trilogy on loss almost entirely to an exploration of mourning related to death.

This book is concerned exclusively with loss of health in adults, and we shall therefore confine ourselves to Bowlby's observations about adults. Bowlby (1980: 181) postulated that the circumstances of the death have significant implications. Thus, relevant circumstances include: (1) whether and to what extent the death was preceded by a prolonged period of nursing care given by the bereaved; (2) whether the death followed upon distortion or mutilation of the body of the deceased; (3) how information of the death reached the bereaved; (4) what the relations were between the deceased and the bereaved during the weeks and days immediately prior to the death; and (5) on the face of it, to whom, if anyone, was responsibility assignable. These five factors determine the grieving process, that is, whether mourning would follow a complicated rather a normal course.

In addition to these five factors, Bowlby examined what he called 'the conditions affecting the course of mourning': (1) the identity and the role of the person lost; (2) the age and sex of the person bereaved; (3) the cause and the circumstances of the loss; (4) the social and psychological circumstances affecting the bereaved about the time of and after the loss; and (5) the personality of the bereaved, with special reference to his or her capacities for making love relationships and for responding to stressful situations. In addition, personality factors and childhood experiences of loss were recognized by Bowlby as essential to understanding individual responses to loss.

Bowlby created a conceptual framework for exploring loss and grief that has since served as a blueprint for research and clinical work. For its sheer depth and breadth, the influence of Bowlby's work is easily detectable in any study of loss and grief. It was the point of departure for another English researcher in grief, Colin Murray Parkes.

Is the process of grief and mourning in many diverse situations involving loss of health analogous to the death of an intimate? This is the most critical question that we shall endeavour to answer in this volume. Bowlby's total preoccupation was with the disruption and eventual loss of a valued relationship. His analyses did not extend beyond the central loss of a loved person, whether that be a temporary disruption in the child-mother relationship in varied situations or the loss through death of a loved one. Murray Parkes extended Bowlby's analyses to determine that loss and mourning was more pernicious in that the reaction to the loss of anything that compromised one's sense of well-being could follow a parallel course to reaction to the death of a loved person. In short, loss and mourning have a much wider application than separation from and/or death of a significant person.

Murray Parkes's research into bereavement has confirmed that any significant loss, regardless of its source, has the potential for creating an analogous pathway for grief and recovery comparable to the reaction to death. In his well-known study of psychological responses to amputation, Parkes was able to show that the common elements of reaction to bereavement are: (1) a process of realization, that is, the way in which the bereaved moves from denial or avoidance of recognition of the loss towards acceptance; (2) an alarm reaction – anxiety, restlessness, and the physiological accompaniments of fear; (3) an urge to search for and to find the lost person in some form; (4) anger and guilt, including outbursts directed against those who press the bereaved person towards premature acceptance of the loss; (5) feelings of loss of internal sense of self or mutilation; (6) identification phenomena – the adoption of traits and mannerisms, or symptoms of the lost person, with or without a sense of the presence of his self; (7) pathological variants of grief, that is, the reaction may be excessive and prolonged or inhibited to emerge in distorted form.

Having identified these common elements of grieving, Parkes noted that prima facie it was hard to compare the loss through death of one's wife with the loss of a leg through amputation. However, as his own research and more contemporary investigations show, the pathways followed by a person grieving the death of his wife and a person grieving the loss of his leg have more in common in their efforts to come to terms with the loss than might at first appear to be the case.

First, we shall summarize Murray Parkes's findings of the Amputation Study. Parkes posed the question: Does an amputee, on losing a limb, work through a process from denial to acceptance of the loss of that limb? His answer was, 'Yes.' His research showed that 39 per cent of amputees in his study had an initial reaction of numbness, while all forty-six of his subjects experienced the presence of the limb following amputation. Quite strikingly 86 per cent stated that they often forgot that they had lost a limb. A year later, 80 per cent still had some sense of the presence of the limb (since Parkes's research on the topic of phantom limb during the 1970s, much progress has been made to unravel the mystery of this seemingly inexplicable phenomenon) and 46 per cent found the loss of their limb to be still unbelievable.

Remarkably, Parkes also discovered what seemed to him to be parallel processes of grieving whether the loss be one's own limb or a person who had died. In addition to the sense that the amputated limb was still there (phantom limb), many of the amputees he studied showed other signs of bereavement during the first year following the amputation, such as feelings of anxiety, loss of appetite, weight loss, and sleep disturbance. Some 63 per cent of his subjects expressed concern about the way their limbs might have been disposed. Parkes tells the story of a man who had a clear view a chimney from his hospital ward, and whenever he saw smoke coming out of the chimney, he wondered if his amputated leg was burning, but he comforted himself by thinking that his leg might have been preserved for medical research. This process is not entirely analogous to searching for the deceased by the bereaved, yet there are interesting similarities.

Further similarities in the grieving process of the two groups were to be found in their pining for the lost object. The amputees, like the bereaved, were constantly reminded of the world which was no longer theirs. The amputees felt envious of others who had not experienced physical mutilation, the same way a widower might be envious of a couple still intact. These feelings were coupled with feelings of internal loss which meant that they felt incomplete. On the basis of these analyses, Parkes concluded that 'the psychosocial transition from being an intact person to being an amputee is a painful and time-consuming process which is, in many ways, is similar to the transition from married person to widow or widower' (1973: 220). In his analyses, Parkes was able to show that grieving is grieving. The

Table 1
The Parallel Process of Grieving: Loss of Wife and Loss of a Limb

Death of a Spouse	Loss of a Limb
1 Movement from denial to acceptance	1 Same process is observable in amputees
2 An alarm reaction: anxiety, fear	2 Common reaction in persons about to undergo surgery
3 An urge to search for and find the deceased	3 Missing the limb and pining to run or swim; concerns about the disposal of the limb
4 Feelings of internal loss of self	4 Great sense of loss and of feeling different
5 Identification phenomena	5 Phantom limb or presence of mannerisms, etc.; adoption of symptoms prior to surgery
6 Pathological variants of grief	6 Same is observable in amputees

various elements of grieving in reaction to a major loss are similar, whether it be a loss through death, loss of one's limb, or even loss of one's habitual residence through relocation. Table 1 summarizes Parkes's parallel process of grief as associated with the death of one's spouse and the loss of one's limb.

Parkes's contribution was not only an extension of Bowlby's conceptualization of loss, but it further revealed the underlying process of grieving that broadened the basis of the original formulation of object loss. It may not be an exaggeration to suggest that Parkes has laid the foundation for the development of a general theory of grief. These early observations by Parkes have been confirmed and reconfirmed by research. Harvey, in 1996, observed that there are many kinds of losses. These may include the loss to death of biological parents whether early or late in life, the loss of health as a result of disease or injury, the loss of home because of poverty, the loss of contact with friends because of relocation, the loss of peace of mind, resulting from wartime trauma or victimization stemming from domestic abuse or crime. Comparing Parkes's analyses of the elements of loss, not all losses noted by Harvey meet the criteria set by Parkes. Loss of a friend because of relocation, it can be argued, is qualitatively different from loss of a limb or the premature death of a parent. In the following section we shall review two divergent physical losses, namely, loss of a limb which is visible, and hysterectomy, which is an invisible loss of internal organ(s).

GRIEF AND THE LOSS OF A LIMB

Since Parkes's seminal work on grief related to the loss of one's limb, much work on the psychological aspects of amputation has made its way into the scientific literature. This body of literature corroborates directly and indirectly Parkes's proposition of amputation as being a major loss with somewhat differing consequences from individual to individual. On a variation on the theme of amputation of one's leg, Fukunishi (1999) examined the relationship of physical factors, including physical functioning and loss of body appearance, to prevalence and severity of post-traumatic stress disorder (PTSD) symptoms in male versus female patients with burn injury (BI) or digital amputation (DA). Female subjects either with BI or DA exhibited PTSD symptoms, in particular avoidance and emotional numbing. An interesting aspect of this finding was that the reaction of these women whether to burn injury or digital amputation was independent of the severity of the actual burn or number of fingers amputated. This study is of particular interest as (1) it focused on the disfigurement aspect of injury, and (2) it found that even digital amputation, which by any measure may be viewed as less debilitating than loss of a limb, had a profound impact.

Unlike the previous study which found women to be more vulnerable, Laatsch and Shahani found that both younger and male patients tended to show psychiatric symptoms more frequently. In a 1996 study of forty-eight rehabilitation patients, which included a variety of conditions including amputation, they observed an inverse relationship between age and reported emotional distress.

Psychiatric consequences related to the amputation of a lower limb were also reported by Lower (1995). He investigated subjects with cerebrovascular accident or lower limb amputation and compared them with individuals who had had no experience of loss. Depression was a common outcome of loss of a limb or following a cerebrovascular accident. Both these groups also used maladaptive defence mechanisms compared with the control group. No significant differences emerged between the lower limb amputees and the cerebrovascular group. The significance of this study is twofold: (1) psychological maladaptation is a common outcome of serious physical loss, and (2) this experience of serious loss of health appears to have an universal quality regardless of the specifics. This is further confirmation of Parkes's proposition that loss and grief associated with loss of a limb are indeed profound and have complex manifestations.

Loss of a lower limb is more than likely to restrict normal activities. Williamson et al. (1994) investigated 160 amputees in order to assess the impact of the loss of a lower limb on the amputees' lives and emotions. Predictably, more physical restriction and less satisfaction with social contacts was found to be strongly associated with high levels of depressive symptoms. Less use of prosthetics and not sufficient income to meet essential needs were also found to be significant predictors of depressive symptoms. The Williamson study, in a way, addressed what is perhaps the most critical question from a psychological perspective. We should reasonably assume here that the amputation was entirely justifiable on medical grounds. Yet, to reap the benefits of such surgery requires that some essential conditions be met: (1) adjustment to the loss of the limb-restricting activities; (2) satisfaction with the assumptive world; and (3) acceptable financial circumstances. Rehabilitation necessarily requires overcoming the loss of the limb, the use of prosthetics, and participation in activities designed to help patients re-engage with their social world. Failure to achieve success in these aspects translates into debility and isolation. Lack of finances is a source of stress and even distress. Depression and depressive symptoms under those circumstances would appear to be a predictable response.

Alienation, which was explicitly discussed in the preceding study, was one of the central questions investigated by Bhojak, Nathawat, and Swami (1989), in a group of thirty men with lower-limb amputation. Perceived body distortion was common in this population, providing an added explanation for patients' sense of isolation and feeling different. Although this study did not make any direct connection between alienation and distorted body image, at a common sense level it seems logical that a patient's distorted body image would serve as a disincentive to engage or re-engage with the social world.

The value of positive psychological response to surgery was confirmed in an investigation by Dunn (1996) of 138 persons with lower-limb amputation. Patients who found positive meanings in the surgery, and perceived control over their disability also showed lower levels of depression. This study offers an antidote to the previous two which showed the negative responses of the patients to the loss of limb. If the surgery is viewed not only as a medical necessity, but as having had some personal value, then the sense of loss is significantly mitigated.

TWO CONTRASTING CASES: MR ABRAMS AND MR BASSETT

Our clinical observations of working with amputees both at the preoperative and post-operative stages tend to bear out many of Parkes's observations. Mr Abrams, about to undergo disarticulation of his arm from his shoulder, was seen standing in front of a mirror holding his offending arm behind his back, trying to imagine just what it would 'look like once the arm was gone.' This man was fully engaged psychologically with his potential loss. In his mind, he stated, he could not begin to imagine life without his arm. His level of distress was very high indeed as the date of his surgery approached. Anyone observing him would have concluded that he was in the throes of deep mourning.

In contrast is the story of Mr Bassett, whose inability to comprehend the nature of his impending loss (below-the-knee amputation of his left leg), which could be interpreted as denial, led to very adverse consequences following the surgery. Aged 64, Mr Bassett had a prolonged history of diabetes which eventually culminated in the below-knee amputation of his left leg. On his admission to hospital for this surgery, he maintained a cheerful outlook. He, in fact, seemed oblivious of the gravity of his surgery, and his almost total lack of anxiety was striking. When seen by a young psychiatric resident for preoperative psychiatric evaluation, the patient gave no evidence whatsoever of any concern. This resident was very impressed by the 'positive' outlook of this patient, and reported his findings to the supervising psychiatrist.

One obvious question was about Mr Bassett's almost total absence of anxiety either about the surgery or its aftermath, and how one might explain it. The resident's response was that the patient was so relieved at the prospect of a pain-free existence that loss of his leg seemed to this man to be nothing short of a blessing. Questions were raised about the defence mechanism Mr Bassett seemed to be employing. Was he, in fact, in denial? This is an important consideration. How concerned should one be about such total absence of anxiety?

Further investigation into this patient's past revealed some startling facts. The most telling concerned his career as a professional football player of some repute. Mr Bassett had achieved national recognition through his physical ability. The symbolic meaning of the loss of a leg for a star football player could hardly be overlooked. Perhaps, his almost nonchalant attitude to the surgery was explicable in this way. Loss of a leg, almost under any circumstance, is a trying experience, and in reaction fear, anxiety, and even anger may be anticipated. For a man whose legs played such a huge role in his success, the prospect of losing a leg is analogous to a singer losing her voice. In view of the enormity of this loss, his recourse to denial made sense.

Mr Bassett's grieving did not begin until well into his rehabilitation. He was, to begin with, very angry and non-compliant and showed little interest in the rehabilitation program. Over time, however, his anger gave way to sadness, and it was only then that he could embark on the path of recovery. This case is not a straightforward tale of loss and grief. Rather, it is an illustration of the varying levels of investment patients may have in their limbs, and how the loss of one of them, might shape individual responses. The other point of note is the ease with which response or more precisely lack of response to the potential loss could be misjudged even by a competent clinician. Recovery simply cannot commence without a clear acknowledgment of the loss, and then travelling through the grieving process.

HYSTERECTOMY

Loss

Hysterectomy, which results in the loss of the uterus and ovaries – invisible reproductive organs – tends to generate a wide range of emotions in women. As this selected review will reveal many women react to their loss of reproductive capacity with depression, loss of identity, and varying levels of grief. Raphael (1982) described hysterectomy as a 'crisis of loss.' She noted that sadness was common, which reflected grief over the loss of body parts, loss of childbearing capacity, perceived loss of attractiveness, and 'perceived loss of some core aspect of feminine self.' She found that some 30 per cent of subjects developed depression, another nearly 25 per cent general health impairment, and 16.5 per cent reported deterioration in sexual function after hysterectomy.

In a comprehensive review of the literature on reproductive loss Dupuis (1997) found that losses associated with hysterectomy were experienced at two levels. First, there is loss of the fantasy of having a child and being parents. This particular loss, related to parenthood, is clearly a function of age. Second, there is loss of status associated with a perceived change in the identity of the patient, a sense of loss of control, loss of sexual spontaneity, and loss of self-esteem. Of course, loss of self-esteem is inextricably tied to the realization that this surgery fundamentally altered the very nature of womanhood. Many of these losses were not necessarily rooted in reality, but rather they reflected the inseparable nature of womanhood with the capacity for reproduction. Any insult to the capacity to reproduce thus goes to the very root of many women's identity.

This particular theme, that is, hysterectomy being an assault on the identity of the woman, was analysed from a feminist-poststructuralist perspective by Dell and Papagiannidou (1999). Their analysis was based on the transcripts of ten Greek women who had hysterectomies followed by oophorectomies for benign conditions. These authors argued that in a patriarchal society women's body was pathologized as uncontrollable. For others, the surgery denoted absence of control and loss of femininity. Yet for some women, hysterectomy was a kind of liberation, and offered resistance to the patriarchal discourses which regarded privileged women with reproductive capacity as complete and sexual. This point of view is an attempt to show the political and cultural influences on our value system, and offers a refreshing alternative viewpoint, that is, loss of reproductive function is not only not a loss, but could be a liberating experience and that to be a woman meant much more than the capacity for childbearing.

Nevertheless, study after study continues to provide further confirmation about the profoundly negative effects of hysterectomy on women's psyche. In a relatively early study involving thirty-seven African-American women who had had a hysterectomy, Bernhard (1985) discovered four areas of fears and concerns: (1) personal physical attractiveness, (2) loss of womanhood, (3) ability to engage in sexual activity, and (4) partner's response. Bernhard carefully pointed out the value of education and accurate knowledge about the anatomy and physiology of the reproductive system, wound healing, and sexual responses. Such knowledge not only hastened recovery, but considerably reduced suffering and insult associated with this surgery. The value of education was also noted by Ananth (1983). His study showed that women under thirty years of age, childless women, and those having infrequent intercourse were more vulnerable to psychological distress. He recommended sexual counselling.

Steiner and Aleksandrowicz (1970) observed that loss of uterus set in motion a process analogous to mourning. They focused on the fears of mutilation of the uterus. This study predates Parkes's formulation of the grieving process as being connected with losses other than the death of a loved one. The phenomenon of mourning re-emerges in the literature in a paper by Roeske (1978) who claimed that 'a mourning process occurs as a woman reintegrates her gender identity,' thus lending further credence to the prevailing notion that loss of the uterus is indeed perceived by the woman as an assault on her identity.

That loss associated with hysterectomy is neither inevitable nor universal was the finding of a study by Roopnarinesingh and Gopeesingh (1982) of upper-class West Indian women. For many of these women hysterectomy represented loss of femininity, loss of reproductive potential, and loss of their husband's attention. Nevertheless, of the 100 subjects, ninety-two stated that they did not regret the operation. Despite their reservations, they did see the medical need for their surgery. These authors, however, were less than convinced of the value of this surgery for women below the age of 40. A more recent study also reported that the consequences of hysterectomy on body image and sexual dysfunction exerted only very limited effects (Anderson and LeGrand, 1991). Furthermore, body image remained stable following the diagnosis and treatment of the disease.

This brief and selected review of the literature leaves little doubt that for many women loss of their uterus is a source of grief. Reasons for that are many and complex. One explanation suggested earlier in this section is to be found in societal attitudes towards women, and the value placed on their reproductive capacity. This perspective cannot be meaningfully separated from the individual suffering experienced by many women undergoing this surgery. Almost all studies tend to confirm that a woman's identity is tied to her reproductive capacity, and its loss is then unfortunately equated with loss of identity. With hysterectomy loss of reproductive capacity must be viewed as the central loss, as all the other losses such as fear of loss of sexuality or decline in marital satisfaction emanate from this compromised sense of self. We shall discuss the question of the loss of identity associated with chronic illness in a subsequent chapter. We hope that the key point that this review has been able to make is that loss of an invisible organ is capable of engendering much grief and sorrow, not unlike the grief and sorrow we associate with bereavement.

Depression

The preceding review gave us a sense of how the loss of her uterus leads a woman to what may be termed as 'normal grief.' This section will expand the reaction to hysterectomy to include atypical grief which often manifests as psychiatric problems, mainly depression. In the chapter that follows, we consider the question of the many and diverse reactions to loss that deviate from the natural or normal process of grieving. This section serves as a prelude.

Even a quick perusal of the hysterectomy–depression literature brings to the fore the body of evidence that has shifted over the years from depression being a relatively common outcome of hysterectomy to a clear rejection of any such inevitability.

Cohen, Hollingsworth, and Rubin (1989) complained that, although understanding of the physiological complications of hysterectomy had changed markedly over the past several decades, no such change was evident in the understanding of the psychological and psychiatric complications. They noted that hysterectomy was linked to the near-inevitability of depression in every major textbook, despite the fact that research had, by and large, rejected any such connection.

Two studies attest to the difficulties of making any direct link between depression and hysterectomy. Lalinec-Michaud and Engelsmann (1988) compared 152 women undergoing hysterectomy with 72 women undergoing other gynecological procedures. Depression was assessed before and after surgery. Depression in both groups was associated with past history of depression and lower education. For the hysterectomy group, fears related to changes in sexual life and the spousal relationship emerged as important factors contributing to depression. The authors concluded that the 'inner representation' of hysterectomy played a role in the development of depression. What remained unclear from the study, however, was whether these women were clinically depressed or going through mourning their perceived identity change.

In a separate report on the same study, Lalinec-Michaud, Engelsmann, and Marino (1988) reported that depression scores for all groups of patients declined after a year and that the hysterectomy group did not differ significantly from the other groups on their pre- and post-operative depression scores. The significance of these findings is that there is no added or inherent risk for depression for patients undergoing hysterectomy compared with those undergoing other gynecological procedures.

In their study, Turpin and Heath (1979) questioned the high prevalence of depression associated with hysterectomy. They observed that depression after hysterectomy was more a function of reaction to organ loss rather than to the procedure itself. This proposition is more analogous to the process of loss and grief rather than depression. Kav-Vaneki and Zakham (1983) found that depression in post-hysterectomy patients was related to altered self-image, that is, feeling less feminine, and it seemed unrelated to the procedure itself. Bhatia et al. (1990), in a study of Indian women, reported a variation on this theme. They found that the depression score for fifty women who underwent hysterectomy was high in the early post-operative phase, but declined significantly after four weeks. Marital and social adjustment either remained unchanged or improved. The conclusion was that depression, while common, was only a transient problem.

Symptoms associated with active mourning overlap with depressive symptoms. This is well known, but not addressed in this literature. The suggestion in many of these studies is that depressive symptoms, although common, could also be explained from the perspective of a compromised sense of self that many of these women reported.

A CASE EXAMPLE: MRS CLIFF

The story of Mrs Cliff encapsulates many of the problems experienced by hysterectomy patients. This was a woman with a long history of marital problems that included general disaffection and serious sexual conflict. Her gynecological problems presented as pelvic pain, and she was diagnosed with endometriosis. At that time, the treatment options were more limited and confined to the contraceptive pill or medication like danazol which had serious masculinizing effects. Mrs Cliff was advised to have a hysterectomy, to which she agreed. The benefits of this surgery were far from evident. The follow-up report suggested that she was no happier after the surgery, sexually things were no different, and in her mind the surgery had simply failed to deliver what she had expected. A noteworthy aspect of the case was that Mrs Cliff's sense of womanhood was not in the least compromised by this surgery. Rather, she was disappointed with the medical profession for subjecting her to what she judged to be a useless surgical procedure.

This brief case report corroborates some of the research findings that pre-morbid personality and ongoing life issues tend to influence a person's reaction to loss. Surgery did not ameliorate Mrs Cliff's pain, nor did it solve her sexual problems. Surgery, in short, was not the answer to this patient's marital and social problems. She showed no obvious signs of grief, but rather disillusionment that the surgery had failed to deliver the results she had hoped for. Perhaps, Mrs Cliff's expectation of what benefits may accrue from the surgery was unreasonable. Research findings are contradictory in relation to satisfaction with sexual intercourse after hysterectomy; some studies report improvement in sexual functioning, while others fail to find any change (Ferroni, 1994; Galyer et al., 1999).

CONCLUSION

Do some women develop a major depressive disorder after a hysterectomy? The answer has to be in the affirmative. Nevertheless, the weight of the evidence suggests that, although many of these women experience high level of distress, (1) the actual prevalence and incidence of depression is difficult to assess, and (2) the issue of real and potential loss associated with hysterectomy looms large in the minds of many women undergoing this procedure.

One way or another, hysterectomy seems to carry the potential of inflicting great damage to the very identity of a woman. Loss is inherent in that notion. As Dupuis (1997) noted there are many losses associated with infertility and hysterectomy which often lead to profound feelings of grief. Other losses experienced are the inability to be a parent, loss of status (in the eyes of society), a sense of loss of control, loss of sexual spontaneity, and loss of self-esteem. The nature of this loss does not readily lend itself to common sense unless certain conditions are added. A very major consideration is the age of the woman, and the circumstances that led to the surgery. For example, depression was found to be more common in patients undergoing emergency hysterectomy than in patients whose hysterectomy was a non-emergency surgery (Lalinec–Maced and Engelsmann, 1985). Hysterectomy as a consequence of cancer is more than likely to bring a sense of relief to a patient, and not grief. This surgery removes a woman's reproductive capacity. This is the most pronounced loss. Hence, surgery may be differently interpreted by women of different ages. There is very little direction to be found in this respect in the literature.

There appears to be a fair degree of agreement that the feeling of loss of femininity is widely reported by women after a hysterectomy. Perceived loss of femininity then becomes a focal point of loss and grief. Some studies suggest that the sense of loss does not set in for a period, and then it manifests as depression; others report that many women experience grief almost immediately following the surgery, while some even have apprehension about loss of sexuality, changes in marital relationship, and loss of femininity before the surgery.

Without the benefit of a detailed study of the mourning process associated with hysterectomy, it is difficult to speculate about the pathway that reaction to this particular loss may follow. From a clinical perspective a critical question concerns the nature of recovery. The literature seems to suggest that grief, although common, is short-lived, and depression is far from inevitable in women after a hysterectomy. Nevertheless, in the absence of any longitudinal studies tracking the mourning process, it is hard to assess what proportions of such patients experience grief and go through 'normal mourning,' and who and how many may embark on the path of 'atypical grief.'

To state the obvious, loss and grief are an inherent part of life. This subject was comprehensively and scientifically investigated by Bowlby, whose contribution to this field of study remains seminal. Parkes expanded on Bowlby's perspectives, and through research and clinical observations demonstrated the similarities in the grieving process regardless of the object of the grief, whether death of a loved one or loss of a limb or any other kind of loss significant to the mourner. The grieving process tends to follow similar pathway, which, generally speaking, leads to recovery. Nevertheless, this process can go very wrong, leading to atypical grief or even mental illness.

We have tried in this chapter to show the loss and grief associated with two very different types of surgery: loss of a limb, usually a leg, and hysterectomy, which deprives a woman of her reproductive ability. Research with amputation seems to confirm Parkes's contention that the grieving process observed in amputees is analogous to the grieving process that begins with the death of a loved one.

Such information is not available with hysterectomy patients, and research findings are ambiguous. Psychosocial factors are major determinants of individual response to this surgery. The societal value, real and perceived, of women as reproductive agents can and does negatively influence a woman's attitude. Age is another critical factor. For post-menopausal women the possibility of reproduction does not exist, although sexual issues remain important. When the reason for the surgery is obvious – for example, when it is for malignancy – women respond positively to hysterectomy. The notion that depression is an inevitable consequence of this surgery has been firmly laid to rest. Research has not clarified the origins of this myth. Perhaps, they lay in a belief, in a patriarchal society, that insult to the very womanhood of a woman as a result of this surgery was so enormous that psychiatric illness was a predictable outcome.

It remains undeniable that loss and grief are commonly associated with mutilating surgery, whether the body parts involved are visible or not. Psychological and psychosocial assessment at the preoperative stage may yield great benefits for these patients. During such an assessment, many myths associated with the surgery can be dispelled, and interventions based on psychological findings can be planned.

2

Loss, Sadness, and Depression: Many Faces of Abnormal Grief and Other Complications

In the previous chapter the notion of loss related to health was described both in general and specific terms. We established that loss of a limb or loss of reproductive organs for women, that is, loss of health and functioning, are understandable reasons for the grief that ensues. We also considered the normal grieving process associated with the loss of a limb and the general demythologizing of a strong association between hysterectomy and depression. Yet, loss of health has the potential of producing atypical grief or even psychiatric disorders. The literature on chronic pain shows consistent elevation on the Beck Depression Scale for a significant proportion of such patients, placing them in the category of clinical depression. It is not our intention to revisit the pain–depression debate, but rather to accept that losses associated with chronic illness are capable of causing much grief and even depression.

Atypical or abnormal grief has been the subject of sustained investigation ever since Freud published his seminal work on mourning and melancholia. In more recent times Bowlby and Parkes have furthered our understanding of why and how the process of mourning can go wrong, and create potentially serious challenges for persons unable to find any significant resolution for their loss. It must be noted in this context that while much of atypical grief is generally associated with the death of a loved one, Parkes extended the concept to include other kinds of losses, and his research into the loss of a limb and the associated grief raised the possibility that amputees may experience atypical grief in the face of such a major physical loss. The case of the amputee in the previous chapter raised the possibility that almost total denial of any negative consequences of losing a leg could lead to an atypical grieving process.

The entire field of grief study is undergoing a major re-evaluation. As a preliminary step, a comprehensive definition of loss has been proposed by Miller and Omarzu (1998): 'Loss is produced by an event which is perceived to be negative by the individuals involved and results in long-term changes to one's social situation, relationships, or cognitions.' Loss is thus an interactive process between individual perception, attribution, and the social context. This definition allows for individual differences in responses to loss, and provides a much broader social and psychological base to understand both normal and abnormal grief reactions. Some elements of this approach can be easily detected in the work of Parkes and Weiss (1983) in their investigation of widows.

Losses associated with chronic illnesses tend to happen over time, and do not have the suddenness even of an expected death. The progression of the effects of these losses as experienced by many patients is far less dramatic than the reaction to death, as our case illustrations will demonstrate. The entire process of grieving such losses may have a slow and even an insidious onset, and recovery from such grief is complicated by the changing nature or unpredictability of the course of many chronic disorders responsible for the losses. The notion of proceeding through the stages of grief, as discussed in Chapter 1, in an orderly manner is also put under considerable strain. The very idea of a journey through such orderly phases, given the ups and downs of chronic illness, becomes questionable. Thompson (1998) suggested that there may be a variety of different grief processes and stages. The particular characteristics of any stage of grief that a person may endure will depend on that individual's personality and circumstances might have added, the uncertain nature of any individual's course of a chronic illness. The onset of rheumatoid arthritis in many people is slow, and this disease may remain quiet for many years in some. For others deterioration is rapid, the personal losses involved are enormous, and a complicated grieving process follows. The concept of atypical or abnormal grief requires considerable modification for these reasons to determine whether an individual patient has adapted well to the changes associated with a given chronic illness or whether the struggle continues. At what point might it be prudent to suggest that an individual 'has come to terms' with the illness and the losses involved? Or, when should it be determined whether depression or other forms of psychological problems have emerged to complicate this process? Before we examine the specifics of loss and grief, and indeed how the grieving process can and does go awry with chronically ill patients, we shall briefly consider Parkes's research in this respect.

PARKES AND ATYPICAL GRIEF

First, we shall examine here, based on Parkes's research, some of the general factors that may lead to atypical grief, and second, we shall review briefly Parkes and Weiss's investigation of widows and the reasons for atypical grief in that population. The key question that we hope to answer is whether a general understanding of atypical grief enhances our appreciation of the complicated grieving process we witness in chronically sick patients.

The two lynchpins of Parkes's criteria for atypical grief are (1) prolonged grief and (2) delayed grief. A careful study of his case studies highlights these two phenomena over and over again. The case of Mr Abrams (from Chapter 1) falls into the latter category. A great deal of empirical evidence supports the contention that there is a lessening of the intensity of grief together with recognition of the permanent nature of the loss. A point not often stated is that the bereaved desires to regain control and begin to resume some semblance of normal life. When these factors fail to materialize and there is little evidence after a certain amount of time (the actual amount of time may vary somewhat) that the mourner is still in the throes of deep grieving and showing very little sign of acceptance of the loss, then the grief can be legitimately described as atypical.

Delayed grief, as the term suggests, is a failure to display the emotions that are normally associated with a major personal loss. Individuals delaying their grief carry on as though nothing much has changed. Delayed grief can also be prolonged. In his original work, Parkes found that many patients with atypical grief presented with a variety of psychiatric problems including alcoholism, somatic symptoms, and depression. Depressive symptoms, such as neurovegetative symptoms, guilt, and hopelessness, are commonly seen in bereaved patients. In many patients chronic illnesses and clinical depression coexist, and in many others depression, often prolonged, is more readily attributable to their losses.

On the basis of his research and observation, Parkes developed a set of four categories of predictors for atypical grief. These determinants were a major departure from the strictly intrapsychic view of grief. Parkes considered: (1) antecedents, including factors such as the experience of loss during childhood; (2) the mode of death, whether sudden or prolonged; (3) concurrent factors, such as age, gender, and cultural background; and (4) subsequent factors, such as the availability of social support. In the chronic illness literature, some of these factors have been found to be important in predicting outcome. For example, the value of social support in effectively dealing with chronic illness has been demonstrated over and over again (Thomas and Roy, 1999). Similarly, in a recent study Zautra, Hamilton, and Burke (1999) concluded that fewer positive interpersonal interactions were associated with more avoidant coping and greater reactivity to stressful interpersonal events in a group of fibromyalgia patients. Halberg and Carlsson (1998) in their in-depth review of twenty-two women with fibromyalgia found ample evidence of early loss and other negative events in the histories of these patients which had a profound effect on these women. Childhood abuse has also emerged as an important factor in the genesis of chronic illness and depression (Roy, 1998). Parkes's subsequent research with Weiss (1983) on the recovery process of widows added a critical dimension to the predictors of atypical grief, namely, interpersonal issues. They discovered that women who had conflictual relationships with their partners at the time of the partner's death frequently embarked on a course of atypical grief.

CHRONIC ILLNESS AND ATYPICAL GRIEF

The critical question is the extent to which Parkes's conception of atypical grief or the predictors of grief may be relevant to the grieving process encountered in chronically ill patients. First and foremost, literature on this topic is virtually non-existent. For that reason we shall rely on clinical experience, and attempt to formulate some notion of the atypical grief that we see from time to time in our patients. A generic definition of atypical grief is the inability to come to terms with loss to the extent that there are serious consequences for the patient and his or her intimates. In a subsequent chapter we shall discuss the ultimate price paid by a few patients who committed suicide as a result, in large part, of their inability to come to terms with their loss of health and functioning.

Parkes noted that depression was common in the grieving process. Depression as a manifestation of atypical grief was thus somewhat more hazardous to determine. Yet, in recent years depression as a relatively common accompaniment of chronic diseases has gained considerable currency. Depression as a clinical phenomenon is also much better understood from psychological, biological, and social perspectives even from twenty odd years ago when Parkes published his work. In the following section, we shall visit the question of depression and especially prolonged depression in chronically ill patients as a manifestation of chronic grief.

CHRONIC ILLNESS, DEPRESSION, AND ATYPICAL GRIEF

One of the longstanding debates in the chronic illness literature has centred on the question of whether depression is an integral part of the disease, such as depression and stroke, or depression and a chronic condition coexisting (comorbidity), or depression as a consequence of the losses associated with a chronic disease. Alonzo (2000), in a very thoughtful paper made the following observation, 'The pathophysiology that produces chronic diseases does not begin at symptom onset, and the psychosocial strategies to cope with a chronic illness, whether efficaciously or maladaptive, also do not begin at symptom onset, but develop over the life course.' The importance of this statement in the context of examining atypical grief or, put another way, responding to losses as a result of the illness with prolonged sadness, cannot be overemphasized. In our own observations with patients with problems of intractable pain conditions, the loss of employment or loss of significant roles, which often is the end-result of a deteriorating condition over many years, often is also the beginning of a grieving process with very individualized outcomes.

One of the conceptual problems that has bedevilled research on depression and medical conditions, such as multiple sclerosis, stroke, fibromyalgia, Parkinson's disease, and so on, is the overlapping nature of many symptoms, which make it virtually impossible to separate the two phenomena. We shall briefly address that question as it has implications for sorting out psychological responses to the disease from the disease itself. Also as Bruce (1999), in his analyses of the complex nature of the depression–disability relationship, aptly put it: by no means does every person with a physical disability become depressed or every person with depression become disabled. The level of disability combined with the psychological and social variables may account for the resiliency in some individuals and the lack of it in others. Furthermore, Williams (1998) has offered a critique of the concepts and measures applicable in depression as experienced in chronic pain populations. William's central objection was that psychiatric models have often been inappropriately applied. Uncritical use of measures standardized for populations from which individuals with medical problems had been carefully excluded, and on which chronic pain patients preferentially endorsed somatic symptoms, contributed to these problems.

Randolph and associates (2000) investigated the relationship between multiple sclerosis with depression. They found that neurovegetative symptoms were differentially associated with depression, fatigue, and physical disability. Only one symptom, loss of interest in sex, was uniquely associated with depressed mood. All the other neurovegetative symptoms were associated with both depression and fatigue, but not with physical. disability. Depression as a reaction to illness and disability may not be all that self-evident.

The double-edged nature of the pain–depression problem was addressed by Verma and Gallagher in 2000. They noted that pain and depression may result from poor outcome of the pain disorder itself or that depression might magnify the negative effects of the pain disorder. They were, however, careful to observe that the fluctuating course of a chronic pain disorder and complications such as physical impairment, disability, and loss of role functioning were critical factors in shaping a patient's emotional reaction to chronic pain.

In their investigation of 277 patients with arthritis, Vali and Walkup (1998) reported that a high level of disability is a contributory factor to depression. They removed the somatic items, in measuring depression, and nevertheless found evidence for an additive impact of depression on one measure of disability: days of restrictive activities. Another study, involving twenty-six first-time stroke survivors, reported that nearly two years after their discharge from hospital, they saw themselves as less interested, capable, and independent, and less in control, satisfied and active (Ellis-Hill and Horn, 2000).

Both studies, although examining very different populations, confirm that physical limitation with all its implications seems to be a major factor in producing sadness, hopelessness, and even depression. And at times, depression for some of these individuals takes on a life of its own and sets them on a course that truly resembles atypical grief. This grief centres on things lost and on promises unfulfilled. These individuals remain generally unresponsive to antidepressants, although they may respond well to psychotherapy. Reed (1999) measured the efficacy of grief therapy in reducing these symptoms and increasing overall well-being for individuals with chronic pain and depression. Reed's findings supported the proposition that grief therapy is effective in increasing overall well-being and the chances of returning to work. Underlying this research was the premise that unremitting grief was a relatively common experience of many chronically ill patients.

In the following sections, we shall discuss four cases to illustrate the complex nature of the grieving process that can emanate from the experience of losses. In the first case, we hope to show how unresolved grief translated into unremitting headaches, and how the resolution of grief significantly reduced the headaches. The second case illustrates the importance of the antecedents of grief in individual confronted with persistent, but not very serious health problems, who succumbs to chronic sadness. The third case is of a man who experienced major losses within a very short period: as the result of an automobile accident he suddenly went from being fully functioning to being physically disabled. His grief reaction was prolonged, but understandable. The final case illustrates the critical borderline between chronic depression and chronic grief.

GRIEF AND PAIN: MRS DAVIES

When in her fifties, Mrs Davies was referred to a pain clinic for unremitting headaches that had persisted for the previous six or eight months. Her headaches were described as 'mixed' type, which is a combination of migraine and tension headaches. She had failed to respond to medication including antidepressants. Her headaches were said to be interfering significantly with her day-to-day life.

On close examination of her personal history a number of rather startling facts emerged, the most telling of which was the sudden death of her husband as a result of a myocardial infarction some two years before. In fact, he died virtually on the doorstep of their house as he was making his way from his car to their house. Mrs Davies described this event without much display of emotion, and it took several more sessions before a more coherent story emerged.

Mrs Davies had been married for over twenty years and had a son and a daughter. She could not remember a time when she was without a headache. These headaches interfered with their social life, and beyond that there were occasions when she was not able to do even simple household chores. Her husband was very understanding and never complained. Yet, they had major differences of opinion on child-rearing. She described her husband as easygoing and a very poor disciplinarian with the children. She believed in strong discipline, but all her efforts were 'sabotaged' by her husband. Eventually, she disengaged herself from any effort to discipline the children. She bore an extraordinary amount of resentment towards her husband for undermining her authority with the children. She was raised in a highly disciplined household where children were seen and not heard. Her father made sure of that. Her mother was the opposite. She was kind and gentle, but usually gave in to her father to maintain peace in the family.

When Mrs Davies's husband died so dramatically, her reaction was one of shock and disbelief. However, she recalled being more angry than sad in those early days after his death. That anger persisted at the heart of which was the question 'How could he leave me with all these responsibilities?' Above all, was the responsibility for two teenaged children who had little or no regard for her. This anger became persistent. She remembered crying during the funeral, but not because she was sad, rather she said, because they were tears of anger. Nearly two years after her husband's death, the dominant emotions she showed were anger and dismay. In the meantime, her headaches had become worse, her son was in a hit-and-run accident, for which he was convicted, and the daughter, now a young adult, was housebound. In essence, Mrs Davies's assumptive world was in a state of collapse, and her dead husband was responsible for all of it. She was betrayed by her husband and her sense of betrayal was palpable. Following her husband's death, Mrs Davies saw her family physician on many occasions, mainly with the complaint of worsening headache. Headache, of course is one of the most common reasons for visiting family physicians (Mantyselka et al., 2001). The physician in turn, tried out many different analgesics without any benefit.

Was Mrs Davies depressed because she had failed to grieve the sudden and totally unexpected death of her husband? Are we witnessing atypical grief in this patient? Is the exacerbation of her headache related, in some ways, to this trauma? One possible way of exploring the question of atypical grief would be judge Mrs Davies's reaction against Parkes's determinants for atypical grief , namely, antecedents, mode of death, concurrent and subsequent factors.

As for antecedents, as far as was ascertainable, Mrs Davies did not experience any significant losses during her childhood. Both her parents died in old age and there was nothing unusual about her grieving her parents' death. Her father was overly strict and never quite satisfied with her school performance, but her mother was the opposite. Mrs Davies's childhood memories were mixed. She did not view herself as abused in any sense of the term. She had no past history of mental illness, although she had a long history of mixed headaches. As for her kinship, she had had a conflicted relationship with her husband. She resented his lax attitude towards child-rearing, which had been a major source of conflict. She also harboured guilt mixed with resentment for having to depend on her husband during bouts of severe headaches. She described her relationship with her husband as 'not very intimate.'

Parkes and Weiss suggested that a conflictual marriage could be a contributory factor to a complicated grieving process. His research provided powerful data in support of that finding. Yet, more recent research has challenged that claim. Carr and colleagues (2000) found that widows who were highly dependent on their spouses, such a Mrs Davies, showed elevated anxiety in comparison with widows who were not so dependent. Their overall conclusion was that grief was not necessarily more severe if the marriage was more conflicted. However, in the case of Mrs Davies, who depended on her husband virtually for every aspect of family life, his sudden death left her in a very vulnerable state. She told this author that she had not as much as paid a bill ever since she got married. The entire picture was made vastly more complex by her headaches which only enhanced her sense of dependency on her husband.

Parkes rightly observed that factors such as whether the death was anticipated or sudden could also influence the grieving process. Mrs Davies's husband died without any previous indication that he might have a massive heart attack. Much is known about the difficulties of accepting sudden and unexpected loss. We shall return to this theme in our consideration of sudden unemployment in Chapter 3. Given Mrs Davies's level of dependence, the sudden death of her husband certainly had the potential for complicating her grief.

As for the concurrent factors such as age, sex, and other issues such as personality and cultural characteristics, two factors deserve attention. First, this was a premature death. Mr Davies was in his mid-fifties. The second issue is her personality. Mrs Davies had learned from her youth to internalize her thoughts and feelings. This was her way of surviving a demanding father. Subsequently, in her own marriage she learned not to express her negative thoughts not just to maintain peace, but in great measure, because of her significant level of dependency on her husband. She was angry with him for her inability to function at a level which would have been satisfactory to her. Guilt played a major role in her reluctance to openly express her disagreement.

The last category of determinants, which included social support, secondary stresses, and emergent life opportunities, is critical to our further understanding of Mrs Davies's dilemmas. With regard to social support, Mrs Davies was completely isolated. She did not have a close friend, and her circle of acquaintances consisted of her husband's workmates and their spouses.

She was not very close even to her only sister. Her life revolved around her family and her headaches.

Mr Davies's sudden death had very serious consequences for their two children. The daughter, who was attending college, dropped out, and the son was charged with drunken driving. He was also involved with a woman considerably older than himself. Mrs Davies was at a complete loss as to what she might do. The children had always gone to their father with their problems, first, because he was generally more permissive, and second, from a young age they learned not to bother their mother because of her headaches. As already noted, the only major source of conflict between Mr and Mrs Davies centred on their children. In essence, there were a great many stressors in her life, but sadly, Mrs Davies was lacking in social support. Fortunately, her financial situation was very satisfactory.

When we add up all the factors that might explain Mrs Davies grieving process going somewhat awry, we begin to develop an appreciation of the role that Parkes's grief determinants may play in complicating grieving. Nevertheless, did Mrs Davies give evidence of atypical grief? Yes, her grief was atypical in one particularly telling way. Although it took Mrs Davies several weeks to open up, in the course of therapy, it became apparent that she had as yet shown virtually no sadness over the death of her husband. Rather, her dominant emotion was anger emanating from a feeling of abandonment. Furthermore, within a week or two of her husband's death, her headaches took a severe turn for the worse, and this eventually brought her to the pain clinic. The following period was characterized by frequent visits to her family physician, who tried every known remedy for headaches, including antidepressants, without any positive outcome. Then the situation with the children almost totally derailed her, and further accentuated her feelings of being betrayed by her husband. When she arrived at the pain clinic, other then her complaints of severe and unremitting headaches, a sense of betrayal and abandonment were the most pronounced emotions that Mrs Davies displayed. The other point of note was that she was barely functioning on a day-to-day basis. She was spending an inordinate amount of time in bed.

This was just two years since her husband's death, and during this period, Mrs Davies had shown little sign of taking charge of her altered circumstances. In fact, she had sunk deeper into detachment. It seemed that she had not truly mourned the death of her husband. Additionally, exacerbation of her headaches, which is a form of somatization, may also be seen as a relatively common reaction among the bereaved. In Mrs Davies's case, it was quite extreme, in that her headaches became her primary focus. On the other hand, given the suddenness and the magnitude of her loss, could she have been expected to be more able to function? An investigation by Derman (2000) into the very question of the length of time widows might take for their grief to diminish established that the level of grief in a group of younger widows, with an average age thirty-eight years, did diminish with time, although not significantly until the fifth to tenth year of their bereavement. Strikingly, grief did not entirely disappear even with the passage of time. This study certainly brings into question the common belief, which arose mainly out of crisis theories, that within a relatively short period of six to twelve months, most individuals come to terms with their loss and resume normal activities. Given the suddenness of Mr Davies's death and all the mitigating factors, even two years may not seem like adequate time for her to come to terms with her vastly altered situation. Yet, the possibility that Mrs Davies had embarked on a tortuous path of prolonged and complicated grieving cannot be summarily dismissed.

In term of the stages of grief, the entire question was put under scrutiny by Wortman and Silver (1989). Nevertheless, even they seem to suggest that for many persons the process of grief begins with sadness and sorrow and ends with some kind of acceptance and recovery. Regardless of the very intricate and desirable debate in the psychological literature on this topic, it is difficult to ignore that Mrs Davies appeared to be a long way from any kind of acceptance and recovery. If one takes a functional view, it is apparent that Mrs Davies, other than carrying out her duties as a patient, was barely meeting any of her multitude of obligations. She was also totally devoid of any enjoyment in her life.

Another critical question is the degree to which Mrs Davies's pre-existing condition of headaches rendered her virtually disabled very soon after her husband's death. One might surmise that her grief and emotional distress found almost purely somatic expression. How common is this? Somatic symptoms are ubiquitous in grief, as well as in depressive illnesses. Headaches in particular and pain symptoms, in general, are common accompaniments of grief and depression, as a whole host of studies attest (Bennett, 1997; Carnelley, Wortman, and Kessler, 1999; Clayton, 1974; Prigerson, Maciejewski, and Rosenheck, 1999; Prigerson, Maciejewski, and Rosenheck, 2000; van Grootheest et al., 1999).

Summary

The propensity for Mrs Davies's grief assuming pathological proportions was significant. Failure to grieve was the hallmark of her case. A highly conflictual marriage, history of chronic headache, a compromised role as a mother, and tendency to internalize feelings together with the sudden death of her husband and subsequent problems with her children could be seen as a combination to thwart normal grief off its course and lead grief to assume pathological proportions. Perhaps, most critically, Mrs Davies had shown little or no sign of sadness, longing, or any of other indications or signals commonly associated with grieving. Her most dominant emotions, two years after her husband's death, were anger and a profound sense of betrayal. This reaction is analogous to Parkes's 'alarm reaction,' which is characterized by anxiety, restlessness, and the physiological accompaniments of fear (Parkes, 1983). Mrs Davies met two of three conditions for pathological grief, as identified by Parkes and Weiss (1983): (1) sudden and unexpected bereavement (as a major precursor for poor outcome); (2) a reaction of anger and/or self-reproach, often associated with ambivalence towards the former partner (associated with poor outcome); and (3) reactions of intense yearning associated with a dependent relationship also associated with poor outcome. This last one was not applicable to her, as she showed little or no sign of yearning.

A final thought on this case is the ease with which Mrs Davies's pain problems could have overshadowed her loss and grief. It was in the pain clinic setting that the problems associated with the death of her husband were identified for the first time. This, despite numerous contacts with healthcare professionals. It simply illustrates that pain and especially severe pain or deterioration of a pre-existing pain condition can deflect experienced and caring caregivers from the underlying issues, even when the issue is as blatant as the sudden death of a husband.

IS THIS ATYPICAL GRIEF? – MRS ERIC

Mrs Eric was referred to a pain clinic for unremitting chest and back pain. Both had become so severe that she was no longer able to work, and at the time of her arrival at the clinic, she was on long-term disability leave. There was no specific initiating event other than her mention of a frightening experience she had over twenty years ago: she was being followed by a man in a car and she ran very fast to lose him. On that occasion she experienced her first chest pain, and that pain had persisted to the present. She was diagnosed with mitral valve prolapse and tried on beta blockers, but without any positive effect. At times her chest pain was severe enough to put her in bed, and she became fearful of any demanding physical activity.

Her back pain had an insidious beginning. More than 25 years ago she was in a motor vehicle accident, and she was in another accident six months later when she was pregnant. There were no apparent lasting ill effects from either accident. Some three years ago she was in a rear-end collision, but again, other than a minor whiplash injury, she was unhurt. However, since that third accident, she has experienced neck pain on the left side, associated with occipital headaches. Sometimes these headaches are very severe indeed.

In addition to her medical problems, Mrs Eric also had a history of affective disorder. Her first episode of depression coincided with the death of her father. It was so severe that she was off work for two years. Her last major episode was in the mid-1990s, and to date she remains on maintenance antidepressant medication. Currently, she has no active involvement with psychiatry.

Mrs Eric's personal history is intriguing. She grew up in a household which was at best chaotic. Both her parents were involved in some form of love entanglements with other partners, and they paid little attention to their daughter. Mrs Eric said her mother was an alcoholic, very domineering, and had prevented any emotional proximity between her and her father. Mrs Eric had been an excellent student, but as the family situation became unbearable for her, she ran away from home in her teens.

Mrs Eric obtained employment at a financial institution, where she stayed until she went on disability leave. She described the period between the ages of seventeen and twenty-two as the happiest in her life. Then, at age twenty-three she married a man whom she described as unfeeling and uncaring. She was unable to recall a single redeeming quality that might have prompted her to marry him. Her only explanation was that 'marriage was the done thing.' Within the very first year of this marriage, she decided that she was in an emotionally abusive situation. Her husband was entirely at the beck and call of his parents, and he would disappear for days without her knowledge of his whereabouts. She learned, over time, that he stayed with his parents on these occasions. The matter came to a head when they had a daughter, and he insisted that the child should be put up for adoption, as he had enough responsibilities without adding the burden of child-rearing. This led to serious conflict which continues to date. There have been numerous separations. At the present time, the husband has moved out and is living with his parents. Mrs Eric showed little or no inclination to seek formal separation and divorce. In the meantime, their daughter has developed a potentially serious illness. Mrs Eric felt almost paralysed to take any action, and found new and novel ways of blaming herself for her misfortune. She frequently took to bed, failed to keep her clinic appointments, and invoked helplessness. She acted quite disabled.

The key point of this case is that it would be virtually impossible to explain her level of disability solely on the basis of her physical condition. The turning point in her general functioning was when she went on disability leave. She was very fearful that she might be required to return to work which, she is convinced, she could not do.

It will be erroneous to think that her physical problems are trivial. Nevertheless, her tendency to give-up, her past history of depression, her failure to terminate a chronically unsatisfactory marriage, her extraordinarily compromised self-esteem, and more recently, her daughter's illness have conspired to create a level of disability and suffering that cannot be solely explained by her physical state. She fully recognizes that not returning to work has serious financial consequences for her. At present, she is barely meeting all her financial obligations. Even so, since going on medical leave, she has adopted a hopeless–helpless position analogous to prolonged grief. There is, indeed, past evidence of such behaviour following the death of her father. The antecedents of grief such as emotionally deprived childhood, a very unhappy marriage, and reaction to a father's death all suggest great difficulty for Mrs Eric to come to terms with her losses.

Does Mrs Eric's response to her loss of health, loss of various kinds of functioning, loss of job, loss of income, and increasing level of physical disability justify her state of chronic sadness that has now continued for two years? Is she in a state of atypical grief? That question poses several challenges. As was noted earlier, chronic illness is not an event, and having a chronic condition may give rise to many events. These happen over time. Curiously, Mrs Eric's medical condition cannot by itself explain the degree of her disability. Only when all the antecedents of her grief and her propensity for mood disorder are taken into account can her general reaction to her losses perhaps become comprehensible. Her condition is analogous to chronic sadness or chronic grief. She has known sadness all her life. She recalled the happiest time in her life in her late teens and early twenties, the period that coincided with leaving home and getting married. It seems highly probable that Mrs Eric is in chronic grief now manifest in various medical conditions.

A CASE OF MANY LOSSES AND RAPID DECLINE: MR FRUM

Mr Frum was in a work-site accident and sustained a back injury. At first, the effects of the accident were not serious. A short time after returning to work, however, he began to experience serious pain to the point that he was unable to continue to work. The basis of his pain problem remained unclear, and there was disagreement among medical experts both as to the cause of the pain and of his reaction to it. Nevertheless, within a few months, he went from being a healthy and fully functioning human being to one who was helpless, depressed, and demoralized. Mr Frum had no prior history of any serious medical problems.

Mr Frum was married and had a young child. His wife worked, and between the two of them they had a substantial income. He was very close to his parents. Mr Frum was a churchgoer, had an extensive network of friends, and belonged to a number of social organizations.

Mr Frum was denied workers' compensation, and in a matter of a month or two the family income had dropped by 70 per cent, putting them in the category of the poor. A great many changes in the family arrangements ensued. The couple's sexual activities had come to a complete halt. The family could no longer afford a child minder. Mr Frum could assume that role, as well as many other domestic responsibilities, since he was home and his wife was out at work. He greatly resented these role reversals. This family had no savings, and with the loss of Mr Frum's income, finding cheaper accommodation became a priority. His pain continued unabated, his mood soured, and there was much tension between him and his wife. His social world simply vanished.

Mr Frum became obsessed with his misfortune. His inability to provide for his family was a source of great shame, and gradually, he lost his capacity for enjoyment. Hopelessness and helplessness were his overpowering emotions, at the root of which was a terrible loss of self-esteem as a man, a father, a husband, and a provider.

A key fact that separates Mr Frum from the previous case is the almost total absence in his history of any powerful predictors of grief. His growing up years were uneventful. He was one of two siblings, and the whole family remained very close. Mr Frum was a good student, and at school he participated in many extra-curricular activities which he had kept up until his accident. Yet, Mr Frum became severely depressed, and in spite of psychiatric and psychological treatments, he remained depressed.

One reasonable approach to understanding grief is to judge Mr Frum's reactions against the magnitude of the losses he incurred. For him to find renewed meaning and reconstruct his identity is likely going to be a long-term and somewhat hazardous undertaking. To go from being a healthy and able person to being an invalid with no income is a long drop, and perhaps viewed from this perspective, Mr Frum's prolonged depression makes sense. Yet, given time, Mr Frum may be able to come to see himself as a survivor or as someone who has learned to cope in the face of adversity. But at the two-year point after his accident, Mr Frum seemed a very long way from realizing such goals. This case raises critical questions about the stages of grief when the losses that one is confronted with require a fundamental redefinition of one's identity.

IS THIS DEPRESSION OR CHRONIC GRIEF? – MS. GILL

Ms. Gill presented at our clinic with a long history of rheumatoid arthritis and dystonia of her neck. Over time she had developed a significant level of disability. Furthermore, she really could not remember a time when she had not been depressed. Her psychiatric report suggested that she had a prolonged history of depression which had by and large remained impervious to treatment. By then, she had become quite critical of psychiatry. Nevertheless, her most recent medication had improved her mood to a measurable degree.

Ms. Gill revealed a long history of suffering. She grew up in a totally chaotic household. Her father was in the armed forces and quite frequently away for long periods. Her mother had various debilitating psychiatric disorders. Ms. Gill was vague about her mother's condition other than to say that her mother was pretty much unable to function. Ms. Gill was the youngest of seven siblings. She was unable to a produce a single happy memory from her childhood, and concluded that she had grown up in a loveless environment. She could not recall a time in her life when she had not been depressed. Despite her home situation, she completed high school, left home, and worked for a telephone company for seven years. For the next few years she moved from job to job and then she developed rheumatoid arthritis and dystonia. Her physical capacity declined rapidly until she was unable to work. She became actively suicidal and received psychiatric treatment in a mood disorder clinic. She attributed her suicidal thoughts to the unbearable pain from dystonia. She lived in fear of this pain and even in the course of her treatment at the pain clinic asserted that if her pain got worse, she would kill herself. In the meantime, she spent much time in bed, and despite repeated efforts to engage her in programs offered at the pain clinic she failed to show up after the initial visit.

Analysis

The point of note about this case is that despite her lifelong history of depression, Ms. Gill had remained a fully functioning human being until she was disabled by her dystonia. Along with the decline of her physical health, her social and financial situation also became precarious. She joined the ranks of the poor.

The task of separating her depression from her grief is virtually impossible since so much of the symptomatology of depression overlaps with grief. Yet, despite her depression, Ms. Gill had remained a functioning human being until the onset of dystonia leading to a significant level of disability. The psychiatric assessment did not address the question of her losses. The psychiatrist recommended a new antidepressant and cognitive therapy.

Ms. Gill was confronted with a debilitating medical condition. Did her past history of depression influence her reaction? On the basis of the information available, any firm conclusion is somewhat elusive. Nevertheless, much of her sorrow and hopelessness and fear could be accounted for just on the basis of her painful medical condition and all the losses that followed. So far, Ms. Gill has only marginally responded to antidepressants which may be viewed as negative evidence for mood disorder. The psychiatric assessment recognized the possibility of an underlying mood disorder but failed to address the question of loss and grief. Perhaps the question of depression or chronic grief is moot, and the only answer is the adoption of a comprehensive approach to treat Ms. Gill.

CONCLUSION

It is worth reiterating that there are qualitative differences between grief associated with a single trauma and grief that we witness in chronically ill patients. One such difference is obvious. Often, there is an absence of trauma and even when a patient, for instance, is forced to give up employment, such an event is not entirely unanticipated. The process of grieving differs in another important respect. As we noted in our case illustrations, because chronic illness is on a continuum and has peaks and valleys, the very idea of the stages of grief from disbelief to resolution and acceptance is brought into question. Many patients deteriorate slowly, others quickly, and most patients have many ups and down before the disease becomes quiescent. The unpredictable nature of many chronic diseases complicates the grieving process.

For those and many other reasons, applying the concept of atypical or abnormal grief becomes challenging and a somewhat uncertain task. If we can momentarily return to our cases, Mrs Davies's headaches, the death of her husband, and the subsequent worsening of her head pain, and an underlying depression were intricately intertwined. Did this represent atypical grief? Probably, as she failed to show any signs and symptoms that are normally associated with mourning.

The case of Ms. Gill is also complex and illustrates how reaction and adaptation to chronic illness is profoundly affected by critical psychological, psychiatric, and interpersonal factors. Chronic sorrow would not be an unreasonable formulation in her case.

In the case of Mr Frum, the speed with which his good fortune disappeared probably bears some resemblance to trauma. He went through an identity shift at an extraordinarily fast pace. From being a worker, father, spouse, and a social being, he was reduced in one short year to an invalid. Common sense would find depression to be an appropriate response to Mr Frum's experience. One might hesitate, in face of the magnitude of his losses and the enormous task of having to redefine himself, to describe Mr Frum's reaction as abnormal.

Ms Gill's case is complex. She is undoubtedly severely disabled by her medical condition and her reaction to it has been one of withdrawal and profound fear and sadness. The most critical point of note is that her lifelong depression did not disable her and she had worked until then and lived a life of her choosing. Her dystonia changed all that. She became both physically and psychologically disabled and has remained so for several years. Would she have reacted differently if she did not have a history of depression, or to what extent was her depression influencing her reaction to dystonia are questions that cannot at present be satisfactorily answered.

The literature of chronic illness has paid little attention to this very critical topic of illness and grief. We are in urgent need of some yardsticks with which to measure what may be a healthy adaptation to loss of health and its concomitants.

3

Job Loss and Chronic Illness:
A Situation of Double Jeopardy

Unemployment in the population with chronic pain disorders is known to be higher than in the general population (Stang, Von Korff, and Galer, 1998; Stratton et al., 1996; Von Korff et al., 1992). Job loss or unemployment is a hazardous event in any person's life. When job loss is the direct consequence of declining health associated with a chronic condition, and an inability to function adequately in a job, then the negative effects of job loss are multiplied several-fold (Jackson, Iezzi, and Lafreniere, 1997). Job loss can be a wholly undesirable event with very unpredictable consequences. In an investigation of the effects of unemployment in a population with chronic pain disorders, Rumzek (1998) found that unemployment produces significant effects on the unemployed person's life. Using complex study design Remzek was able to demonstrate that problems associated with chronic pain in combination with unemployment led to more depression, but not more anxiety than experienced in a cohort of employed people with chronic pain conditions as well as a cohort of employed people without pain conditions.

A landmark Canadian study, revealed that unemployment carries a whole host of negative effects (D'Arcy and Siddique, 1987). Significant differences in health status was found between people who are employed and people who are unemployed. Unemployed blue-collar workers were more prone to physical complaints than were white-collar workers, who were more prone to psychological distress. Unemployed people with low incomes, who had also been the principal wage earners, were the most vulnerable of all. This last finding has special relevance for patients with chronic pain disorders, since they generally tend to be blue- rather than white-collar workers.

In this chapter, we purport to show that unemployment in itself is extraordinarily stressful, and has undesirable consequences in virtually every aspect of a person's life. These consequences may include serious health and psychological problems, family violence, other kinds of family conflict, problems with children, and even suicide. Price, Friedland, and Vinokur (1996), in a superb analysis of job loss and the ensuing hard times, noted the 'cascading' effects of job loss. They stated that 'economic hardships (as a result of job loss) can produce a cascade of stressful economic events that challenge the coping capacities of families and individuals both in the short and long run.' In addition to some of the ill effects of unemployment already noted, Price et al. reported other consequences such as increased risk for traffic accidents, criminal activities, and alcoholism.

We shall first present a brief review of the literature on job loss and (1) grief; (2) health, focusing on depression and loss of self-esteem; (3) family issues, including family violence, and (4) a brief consideration of chronic pain disorders and unemployment. Then we present two cases illustrative of the severe negative effects of chronic illness and job loss. These effects happen over time. Most of the patients in our pain clinic had been able to work for varying lengths of time, ranging from a year or two to even ten years. Job loss resulting from chronic illness is qualitatively different from job loss because of a plant closure or from the sudden loss of employment for other reasons. Although for chronic pain patients, job loss may be to some extent predictable, it is nevertheless traumatic. The main source of this trauma is the meaning – both symbolic and real – that we all attach to our work. Not only is there the loss of income (which in itself is hugely important), but also there is the loss of one's social world, loss of self-esteem, and loss of position and status in the family (which is usually that of breadwinner), as well as a great sense of failure and feeling of being stigmatized. An added reality compounding the suffering of many chronic pain patients is the feeling among many professionals that these patients' inability to work may also be their *unwillingness* to continue to work. At the heart of this difficulty is the prevalence of the view that conditions such as chronic low back pain are not true and legitimate medical conditions, and are substantially driven by psychological factors. Patients suffering from such conditions somehow become 'illegitimate' and their inability to work is viewed with suspicion (Roy, 2001).

The social and personal consequences arising out of unemployment have been the subject of research for nearly seventy years. Jahoda, Lazarsfeld, and Zeisel (1933) argued that work serves many critical functions to a person that are essential to well-being. Job loss results in loss of 'manifest functions,' such as earning money, and of 'latent function,' such as regular activities, a sense of identity derived from the job, and social activities.

JOB LOSS AND GRIEF

One patient, who suffered from a number of painful conditions, described her loss of employment as akin to death. She said, 'Dying can't be any worse than being thrown out of work.' She was a healthcare worker, who tried to work part-time for a while, but finally gave up. Her reactions were complicated. At one level, she blamed her employer for not making any readjustment in her assignment, and yet in some ways she felt that she could not have gone on in any case. Her deteriorating health was truly at the heart of this eventuality. Not being able to carry on in her chosen profession amounted to loss of a major attachment for her. Without an appreciation of the meaning and power of this attachment, the severe reactions to job loss cannot be understood. Severe grief over loss of a role that defines so much of who and what we are, compounded by the assumption of a wholly undesirable role, that of a disabled person, is a common response.

Unfortunately, the literature, although ample on topics such as job loss and depression and job loss and loss of self-esteem, is silent on grief. As for the above patient's reactions, her major struggle was with the process of redefining herself. Although her unemployed status developed over a long period of time (some two years) and was not unexpected, she reacted in ways that have commonly been associated with other kinds of losses, such as the death of a loved one or even loss of a limb. However, it is the loss of a societally and personally valued role that explains at least in part this patient's response. The additional and in some ways unique quality of the job loss is further complicated by the reinforcement of the role of being disabled. Unlike workers who may be laid off and seek re-employment, for many chronically ill individuals that is simply no longer an option. Much of the despair we see in our patients emanates from this reality – the finality of this situation. The permanent loss of employment prospects is an irretrievable loss which demands a redefined sense of one's self or one's identity.

Under these circumstances, it stands to reason that the course of grieving may differ significantly from the 'normal' process. Considering the damage to self-esteem and the preponderance of depression among the unemployed, as our review will show, the task is that much more daunting for chronic pain patients. Unfortunately, losing the ability to work for many patients is also a slow and not so slow descent into poverty. Additionally, there usually ensues a long and unpleasant battle with workers' compensation and insurance companies, as there can be serious challenges to the medical legitimacy of the patient's inability to work (Roy, 2001).

Grief as a concept has been rarely invoked in relation to unemployment. One study that did so involved sixty men who had become unemployed over the previous eight years. More than a quarter of them clearly fulfilled predefined criteria for grief. Several measures of job attachment were found to be significantly related to responses characterizing grief (Archer and Rhodes, 1993). As was suggested earlier, people have significant attachment to their jobs as work fulfils many personal and social functions. Regarding the actual grieving process, it may be reasonable to assume that after the initial shock and other responses, most people find some level of acceptance. This last proposition is simply an extrapolation from the findings of various grief studies that tend to show that at some point most people come to terms with their losses.

Nevertheless, close observation of chronic pain patients reveals time and time again that for many of them arriving at an acceptance of being permanently unemployed and permanently unemployable is qualitatively different from a 'normal' job loss. In many ways job loss is the final confirmation of the worst fear harboured by these people, namely, that they are not very likely to regain one of their most valued roles for themselves. Shame associated with the inability to provide for themselves and/or the family is palpable. Shame is not an uncommon emotion reported by people who are unemployed. In a rather unique study of eighty unemployed men, strong feelings of shame were found in 15 per cent of them, and 10 per cent showed milder forms of shame (Eales, 1989). For the chronically ill, shame underlying feelings of guilt is often apparent, and any additional loss of functioning serves to aggravate these feelings. Desperation that may arise out of such feelings can and does have very far-reaching effects, as our case illustrations will show. In a subsequent chapter, we shall consider suicide among the chronically ill and provide two illustrative cases that show how unemployment can contribute to suicide. For people whose health is already significantly compromised, is loss of work a complicating factor? To answer this question we shall look at the literature.

UNEMPLOYMENT AND CHRONIC ILLNESS: A DOUBLE-EDGED SWORD

Unemployment represents a double-edged peril for all chronically ill patients. This was illustrated in a study by Claussen, Bjorndal, and Hjort (1993) of 270 Norwegians who were among both the long-term unemployed and the chronically ill. Their most telling finding was that a psychiatric diagnosis was associated with a 70 per cent reduction in the chances of obtaining work. One obvious observation is the ubiquitous nature of depression in this population. Combine that with unemployment, and the situation becomes ever more complex indeed, circular: a chronic physical condition leading to depression leading to unemployment leading to depression leading to unemployment. In short, a negative cycle is triggered which may not be amenable to any quick solution. This same study found that the absence of a psychiatric diagnosis increased the chances of re-employment by two- to three-fold times.

Averill et al. (1996) found that of a population of 1,000 patients with chronic pain disorders, 67 per cent were unemployed, thus corroborating the findings of Claussen et al. There was a statically significant association between work-related variables and depression. Averill et al. were firm in their conclusion that there is an association between unemployment and increased depression in people who are chronically ill. In a population of individuals who were already depressed, loss of work accounted for even higher levels of depression.

The circular nature of unemployment and depression was investigated by Hammerstroem and Janlert (1997) in a group of 1,060 Swedish youth. They asked whether poor health led to psychological ill health or vice versa. Unemployment was positively correlated with changes in nervous complaints and depressive symptoms, even after controlling for initial psychological health and various demographic variables. The results were generally supportive of the circularity of the relationship between unemployment and psychological health.

The final study mentioned here on the reinforcing nature of unemployment and depression was undertaken by Viinamaeki, Koskela, and Niskanen (1996). This was a prospective study comparing 118 workers laid off as a result of a plant closure and 136 workers employed at a wood-processing plant. The authors analysed questionnaires sent by mail at six and again at eighteen months after the first group of subjects were given notice of termination of their employment. Depression scores were higher at the initial testing for the unemployed group compared with the employed group and showed a marked increase from baseline scores in subsequent follow-ups. The prevalence of high Beck Depression Inventory (BDI) scores increased during the follow-up among the group of unemployed subjects, confirming unemployment as a powerful contributory factor to depression.

This brief literature review confirms the common-sense proposition that being forced out of work because of declining health has even more noxious effects than people being laid off for solely economic or other non-health-related reasons. Similarly, common sense would suggest that one predictable consequence of job loss is loss of self-esteem.

SELF-ESTEEM AND UNEMPLOYMENT

Understandably there is a preponderance of depression and depressive symptoms among the population of people who suffer from chronic pain disorders, and almost invariably depression goes hand in hand with loss of self-esteem. It seems that this also can be said for people who are unemployed. Depression is common among the unemployed, and more than likely self-esteem suffers when a person loses his or her source of livelihood for reasons beyond his or her control. The literature on self-esteem and unemployment is very limited, as the following review will show.

We might assume that high self-esteem would serve as a buffer or mediator between unemployment and the ensuing strain and stress. Jex, Cvetanovski, and Allen (1994) designed a study to test this assumption. A set of questionnaires that included a specific measure for self-esteem was completed by 195 unemployed and 137 employed persons. Surprisingly, only a rather weak association was found between self-esteem as a moderating effect of unemployment and anxiety. However, among women, unemployment was correlated to high levels of anxiety and depression but only among those reporting low self-esteem. This study failed to show the positive role of self-esteem as a buffer, at the same time confirming the negative effects of low self-esteem in unemployed women. This gender difference cannot be easily explained.

The second study is more in the domain of social psychology. Nevertheless, it has relevance to our discussion. Sheeran, Abrams, and Orbell (1995) tested a social comparison theory involving forty-eight full-time employed and forty unemployed individuals in relation to self-esteem and depression. Past levels of self-esteem were highly predictive of psychological distress among the unemployed subjects, whereas the magnitude of any gap between the ideal self and the perceived real self predicted distress among the employed. Intergroup comparisons revealed self-esteem as the main distinction and predictably, depression was higher in the unemployed subjects compared with those who were employed. From a clinical perspective, this study confirms the general contention that unemployment compromises self-esteem, and that the degree to which it does so rests on the level of self-esteem the person had before becoming unemployed.

The final study considered in this section is one that investigated the power of unemployment to damage self-worth (esteem). In a longitudinal study by Goldsmith et al. (1996) of 1,198 subjects in the labour force, it was shown that self-worth is damaged by unemployment. Furthermore, both complete loss of employment and temporary lay-off are harmful to self-worth. Joblessness compromises self-esteem was the core finding.

These three studies confirm a common-sense proposition that job loss, with its propensity for engendering depression and an assortment of other psychological and social problems, can damage one's self-esteem. A critical point, from our perspective, is that for people with chronic pain disorders, who are people already in a vulnerable state, a further attack on self-esteem resulting from any unemployment that ensues tends to leave a long-lasting effect (Roy, 2001).

UNEMPLOYMENT AND FAMILY ISSUES

Unemployment and Family Violence

The impact of unemployment on the family is far-reaching, indeed. One patient involved in an automobile accident developed multiple health problems which resulted in the dissolution of his business and subsequent bankruptcy. His wife, for the first time in their long marriage, had to go out to work. The hopelessness experienced by our patient as his economic world collapsed around him was very evident. When his wife eventually decided to find employment, our patient developed all the hallmarks of clinical depression. He completely withdrew from his family, and it was in this condition that he appeared at our clinic.

Fortunately, this man did not resort to violence, but as will be illustrated in the case example discussed below, violence is perhaps not an uncommon consequence of job loss. Several recent studies have investigated unemployment and family violence, and the findings are worrisome. In an early review on this topic, Jones (1990), identified a clear relationship between unemployment and child abuse. He offered several explanations. Economic hardship, the decompensating psychological state of the unemployed person's mind, loss of the self as breadwinner and other roles, and any ensuing alcoholism emerged as critical factors that contributed to that person's abuse of a child. A very comprehensive investigation into the risk of family violence following unemployment was conducted in Denmark by Christofferson (2000). That study included all Danish children born in 1973, who had been hospitalized because of abuse or neglect between the years 1979 and 1991, when the children were between six and eighteen years of age. This sample comprised 69,623 children. A number of social and personal factors predicted abuse. Key among them was the father's mental illness, parental criminal behaviour, the mother's alcohol or drug abuse, parental lack of education and vocational training, and the mother's long-term unemployment. The curious aspect of the finding was the weight of the mother's, rather than father's, unemployment. All other findings in this study suggested class as the predictive factor. Poverty and lack of education in combination with unemployment appear to increase the propensity for child abuse.

Unemployment was also found to be a major factor in child abuse in a Finnish study. To investigate both mild violence and severe violence in Finland, 9,000 15-year-old students were asked to complete a set of questionnaires. The response rate was 88.8 per cent. Results revealed that unemployment in a family contributed to both mild and severe violence. The participants who were living with single mothers reported the least violence, which to some extent contradicts the previous study, where unemployed mothers emerged as the major perpetrators of violence. In an Australian study of child abuse in the Aboriginal population, the factors that contributed to abuse were related to low self-esteem, poverty, lack of education and unemployment (Cochrane, 1992).

Alcohol abuse, intermittent employment, less than a high school level of education, and recent unemployment emerged as major predictors of partner abuse in a study by Kyriacou et al. (1999). The abused were 256 women who had been intentionally injured by their male partners. They had among them a total of 434 contusions and abrasions, 89 lacerations, and 41 fractures and dislocations. The sample was drawn from the emergency departments of eight large university-affiliated hospitals. Notably, the risk factors for abuse seem to be very similar for both children and women. In a study of violent deaths in Chicago between 1970 and 1990, based on census data and vital records for seventy-five Chicago communities, Almgren et al. (1998) investigated three types of violent deaths: suicide, homicide, and accidents. Their findings suggest that both homicide rates and accidental deaths could be predicted by high rates of unemployment and the family disruption that followed. Almgren et al.'s study is unique for its scope and breadth, and provides confirmation for joblessness as a predictable contributing factor in family violence, in this instance leading to death.

Unemployment and Family Function

The studies in this brief review have identified a powerful set of predictors for family violence, among which poverty, lack of education, and unemployment appear paramount. This is not surprising. There remains a dearth of information, however, on any association between job loss among white-collar workers and family violence. Studies that do exist show an obvious class bias with abuse being predominant among the poor and the otherwise dispossessed, although we know from the larger literature that family violence cuts across all social classes. Perhaps, more targeted research will reveal what the true pattern is of violence is in families where one or both of the adults are unemployed.

Other Family Issues

The family becomes a victim of unemployment, as unemployment adversely affects many aspects of family functioning (see, e.g., Barling, 1990; Bleich and Witte, 1992; Hanisch, 1999; Hoffman et al., 1991; Lobo and Watkins, 1995; Marotz-Barden and Colvin, 1989; Price, 1992; Starkey, 1996). Unemployment can and very often does lead to damage to the health of the spouse and children (Dew, Penkower, and Bromet, 1991; Jones, 1991; Schliebner and Peregoy, 1994; Christofferson, 1994). Spousal stress rises significantly when one or both partners become unemployed (Clark, 1996; Friedmann and Webb, 1995; Wade, 1999).

We shall present the results of additional studies to further confirm our earlier noted observation that the vicissitudes of living with chronic illness are made enormously more compli-cated by unemployment. No one escapes the pain and humiliation that comes with unemployment as a result of circumstances beyond one's control.

Lobo and Watkins (1995), in an in-depth study of the effects of unemployment on families, found that job loss created considerable disruption to a family's customary living arrangements. Primarily, role reversals were not easily or willingly accepted. Loss of income, of course, often led to material deprivation, and marital conflict over family finances was relatively common. Bleich and Witte (1992) reported an overall decline in the quality of the marriage in these circumstances. Wade (1999) investigated six dimensions of stress caused by unemployment:

(a) marital strain; (b) caregiving strain; (c) paid work strain; (d) work–home conflict; (e) stressful life events; and (f) perceived financial difficulties. Depression and family strain were common in this population. Clark (1996) found that the level of marital discord after one or both partners became unemployed was a function of the prior level of satisfaction with the marriage. However, unemployment is not necessarily a major factor in marital dissolution (Starkey, 1996). Christofferson (1994), who studied the long-term effects of unemployment on children, revealed that violence in the home, being bullied in school, and low self-esteem were relatively common. The literature is, on the whole, unequivocal about the deleterious consequences of unemployment virtually on every aspect of family life. We shall now discuss several cases to show that when unemployment is combined with chronic illness, the results can range from a moderate level of grief to family violence.

A CASE OF NORMAL GRIEF? – MR HILL

Mr Hill was referred to a pain management centre several years after he had suffered extensive injuries as the result of an automobile accident. His pain had become intolerable and his wife was experiencing increasing frustration in coping with his 'whimsical ways.' His past history revealed a hard-working man and a very good provider. The couple has three children. All the children received university education and were set for professional careers. The marriage was satisfactory. One pre-morbid issue of importance was Mr Hill's history of alcoholism, for which he had received treatment, and he saw himself as more or less cured.

Following the automobile accident he was able to work for a short while, but eventually he could no longer function in a white-collar profession, and was placed on long-term disability (LTD). Much of his history had to be carefully reconstructed, as he was already unemployed at the time of his arrival at the pain management centre. His wife was very clear that there were marked changes in his behaviour following upon his job loss. It is important to recognize that Mr Hill had no doubt in his mind that he would never work again. He equated going on LTD with being permanently laid-off. He had become increasingly withdrawn and totally detached from family affairs. He spent a lot of time either in bed or in front of the television, while acknowledging that he was only vaguely aware of the programs he was watching on the TV. The couple's sexual relationship had come to an abrupt end, and their sense of togetherness had suffered greatly. Mr Hill's response to all these difficulties was that the solutions were beyond him.

Another critical aspect of Mr Hill's job loss was the effect it had on Mrs Hill's health. Apart from developing depressive symptoms, Mrs Hill's gastrointestinal problems, which had been dormant for several years, were now serious and required specialist intervention. Following his job loss, Mr Hill's attitude and behaviour towards his disability changed markedly. He became indifferent to his health. Furthermore, he became generally inconsiderate, and his wife complained that there was no way of pleasing him. She could do no right.

The family relationships had suffered. The children, while very sympathetic to their father's plight, generally sided with their mother, and over time virtually stopped talking to their father. The whole situation was like a vicious cycle. The deeper that Mr Hill sank into depression and dejection and erratic behaviour, the more the children and Mrs Hill withdrew from him, adding to his sense of abandonment and demanding more.

Analysis

Clearly, some of the hallmarks of reactive grief are evident in Mr Hill's behaviour. He became withdrawn and uncommunicative. This had the undesirable consequence of removing him from the family. He was sad and depressed, and his behaviour in the eyes of his intimates became irrational and incomprehensible. The children reacted by withdrawal, and Mrs Hill suffered a relapse of her gastrointestinal problem. One point of note is that the family members seemed to underestimate

Mr Hill's reaction to his job loss. His reaction was seen as unreasonable, and family support for his loss was absent.

Job loss in the eyes of Mr Hill's intimates was perhaps a natural progression of his failing health. To them it was not an unexpected event. Being placed on long-term disability (LTD) was the logical outcome. What was there for Mr Hill to be so upset and sad about? Should he not have been pleased that he would no longer have to struggle and still have enough income? From the family's point of view, things could not have worked out any better. Perhaps, even for Mr Hill the loss of his job was not entirely unpredictable. Nevertheless, his reaction was not altogether out of proportion. The fact that he was not happy and relieved only caused the members of his family to be puzzled. The situation was made very complex by their negative reaction. There can be two reasons for the family's reaction. First, as already mentioned, there was Mr Hill's increasingly failing health and, second, was the question of the family's relative financial security. If the job loss had translated into major financial hardship, then presumably the family would have reacted differently. Nevertheless, the family reaction was out of tune and only contributed further to Mr Hill's response, which seemed to be well within the parameters of a normal grief reaction to job loss.

A CASE OF PROFOUND GRIEF: MRS INNES

Mrs Innes (see chapters 4 and 9) was diagnosed with rheumatoid arthritis in her late teens. For several years, the disease remained under control. She finished high school and started working in a veterinary clinic as a veterinary assistant. She loved animals and loved her job. A year before her disease became active, she married a man she had known for several years. For several months, she resisted visiting her rheumatologist. In the meantime, her job was becoming increasingly burdensome to her, until on one occasion she received a mild reprimand from her employer and the week after that was unceremoniously dismissed from her job. The loss of this job held much more meaning for her besides that she had now joined the ranks of the unemployed. Taking care of sick animals was a vocation for her. She owned several horses, enjoyed riding, and spent a lot of time in their company.

Following her job loss, Mrs Innes underwent what amounted to a change in her personality. She avoided any human interaction and cried frequently and, paradoxically, engaged in heavy chores that were not essential. It was in this state that she was sent by her family physician to a pain clinic for psychosocial assessment.

Analysis

To be diagnosed with a potentially debilitating disease is unpleasant at any time. To a young person just embarking on major life events such as work and marriage is likely to be catastrophic. The situation is made significantly more complicated when denial is used extensively to fend off fear of deterioration and disability, as was indeed the case with Mrs Innes. Unfortunately, when her disease reached an active phase, her denial was so strong that she postponed contacting her rheumatologist, although she had known him for many years. But her denial collapsed after her employer fired her from her job for inefficiency, even though he did not know that Mrs Innes's inefficiency was a consequence of her disease.

Mrs Innes was in a state of considerable psychological peril when she lost her job. From the time she was diagnosed with rheumatoid arthritis, she had dealt with it by basically ignoring it. She had engaged in counterphobic behaviour by taking on physically challenging activities, and she behaved as though she were healthy. Her employer, for example, never knew about her illness. Consequently, one of the effects of being fired was a rapid breakdown of her defence mechanisms, which were no longer viable. Mrs Innes was now confronted with the double task of coming face to face with her disease and the loss of a role that she truly cherished. She had lived in hope that her disease would magically vanish.

Mrs Innes's reaction to these twin events had all the hall-marks of acute grief. She not only lost her job, but at the same time she was forced into recognizing her decreasing physical abilities. Sadness, anger, and social withdrawal under those circumstances would be highly predictable. In fact, her family physician concluded that she had developed clinical depression.

Mrs Innes was seen in psychotherapy for eighteen months. In the beginning she could not bring herself to talk about her job loss without crying. It took six months before she began to talk freely about her anger and disappointment and was able to slowly move in the direction of acceptance. The focus of therapy was to help her come to terms with the disease, and more important for her future, to engage in a process of redefining herself. We shall be returning to her case in the next chapter to further discuss the most difficult tasks that chronically ill patients have to undertake in terms of developing what amounts almost to a new identity. By the end of therapy, Mrs Innes had found a new vocation and her disease was under much better control.

This case has several noteworthy features. First and fore-most is the young age at which the patient was diagnosed with rheumatoid arthritis. Second, she was fired from a job for apparently poor performance, but in truth because of her deteriorating health. Third, she was forced into a position of confronting both the harsh realities of her disease and the ineffectiveness of her defence mechanisms. These factors create an optimal situation for a complex grieving process because just the job loss in itself is symbolic of many potential future losses, and coming to terms of living with an uncertain future.

A CASE OF EXTREME REACTION: MR JAMES

Mr James (see Chapter 8) had an extreme reaction to losing his job. He was married and had two young children. He and his wife had emigrated to Canada, where having found a good job he had made a good life for himself and his family. All had seemed well. Then an automobile accident turned his life upside down. Failure to find a reasonable solution to his persistent and severe back pain had made his life intolerable. He became unable to function in his job and his employment was terminated.

Previously a supportive spouse and parent, Mr James had become, as his wife described, a tyrant. He was now exceedingly impatient with his wife and children and this impatience would now quickly turn into verbal and even physical abuse. During a family session, he denied any of these problems and demanded that his back be 'put right.'

The impact of the changes in Mr James had very far-reaching consequences for his wife. From what we could ascertain, the marriage had been quite satisfactory prior to Mr James's accident and subsequent job loss. According to his wife, Mr James had taken on a virtual change of personality. He had severed his engagement with all family activities and become abusive. Mrs James was confronted not only with serious financial problems and added family responsibilities, she now also lived in very real fear of verbal and physical abuse from her husband.

It took some persuasion to bring Mrs James to our clinic, as she was afraid of how her husband might react. She was especially concerned about the well-being of their three young children. She was emaciated, looked depressed, and complained of persistent sleep disturbance, anorexia, and a substantial lowering of mood. She acknowledged that she now lived in fear of her husband and his unpredictable behaviour. She was diagnosed with clinical depression and given appropriate treatment and professional support.

Analysis

Mr James's case exemplifies the notion of the cascading effects of chronic disability coupled with unemployment. From being reasonably well-functioning, this family had become in danger of disintegration. Mr James's transformation was of unexpected proportions. A kind and caring man, on losing his central role in the family, turned on his family members in a manner both vicious and unpredictable. The consequences of Mr James's back problem and loss of employment (it is impossible to separate the two) were unforeseen. He had come to Canada with nothing and managed to establish himself and become a good provider for his family. Losing all that for a reason that he could not fully comprehend goes some way in explaining his dramatic reaction.

Mr James's violence was completely incomprehensible to his wife. She was at a total loss to even begin to understand his behaviour and concluded that he had 'gone out of his head.' She was not far wrong. Mr James felt totally let down, and unfortunately, his remorse found an external expression in violence. Family violence following job loss is not unknown. Yet what was so surprising for Mrs James was the depth of change in her husband's behaviour. As she said, he was now like a stranger to her. Another point to note, as a consequence of Mr James's disability and unemployment, was the effect on his wife's health. Mrs James herself developed a mood disorder. In short, this family was coming apart. All three children were at risk. This case illustrates some of the worst consequences of chronic illness and unemployment.

CONCLUSIONS

To people with chronic illness losing their job is the final affirmation of their identity as being someone who is chronically sick. By the time a patient has reached the stage of becoming jobless or more accurately has become unable to work, many other roles and functions have either already been lost or are in the throes of becoming lost. For a healthy person, unemployment is primarily a loss of work with all its negative effects, but there always remains the hope and the possibility of re-entering the workforce. For the chronically sick, the absence of any hope of ever being employed again makes this experience more difficult and even harder to accept. The psychological, social, and health consequences of unemployment are well documented. When we examine the effects of chronic illness and unemployment, a telling fact emerges: the effects of unemployment are not all that different from the effects of chronic illness. The difficulty, from a clinical point of view, is in trying to sort out the consequences of one from the consequences of the other, in addition to identifying their mutually potentiating effects.

Job loss and chronic pain disorders both adversely affect all family members, as well as family functioning. Health effects on the spouse, frequently depression, often follow in both cases. This should not be surprising in view of the tremendous strain experienced by everyone as they lose what had been their significant and meaningful roles and are forced into having to redefine themselves, as well as their family. Such situations, understandably, leave people prone to depression.

Is the loss of one's job easier to accept when it is a result of illness as opposed to other social and economic reasons? The research literature does not provide any clear answer. Yet, common sense would dictate that for a person who is chronically ill, job loss is pretty much predictable. This happens over a period of time, although as was evident in one of our cases, not always. A point to note is that it is possible to prepare a chronically ill patient for this eventuality, and this may have a moderating effect. Nevertheless, grief and mourning were evident with all our case examples. Grief and mourning are also inevitable when patients with chronic disorders, having already lost their health, lose their jobs – usually forever.

4

Declining Health and Functioning: Redefining Identity

The gradual and cumulative loss of all major sources of gratification, largely associated with the loss of one's perceived roles in life, is the experience of many chronically ill patients. Unlike acute illness, when there is a sudden flight into the sick role, but then resumption of normal activities after a relatively short intermission, chronic illness with its unpredictable vagaries presents almost insurmountable challenges. Some patients do remarkably well in the circumstances, and others fall prey to the only role that remains available to them and that is the role of being chronically sick.

People define themselves in terms of what and who they believe they are. Self-definition is rooted in our ability to live with some sense of balance with our environment. People seek equilibrium between themselves and their environment. This equilibrium is thrown into jeopardy by chronic illness. Our sense of well-being is, to a significant degree, related to our ability to meet our obligations through work, by being good parents and friends, and by being good citizens. These obligations are much harder to fulfil in face of chronic sickness. Although a partner does not cease to be a partner in a relationship when struggling, say, with multiple sclerosis, it can alter the fundamental nature of the partner relationship, the underpinning of which often is reciprocity, beyond recognition. Before considering the literature on this difficult topic, we examine the case of a patient illustrating human resiliency in overcoming the difficulties of living with pain, disability, and with rheumatoid arthritis.

Mrs Innes (see chapters 3 and 9) was diagnosed with rheumatoid arthritis very early in life. Although she had suffered the symptoms for several years, but she had not sought medical help not until they were severe enough to be interfering with her daily living. The disease progressed rapidly from that point, and in barely a few months, Mrs Innes was no longer able to work. Thus began a major crisis for her.

At this point Mrs Innes had been married for just over a year. Until then, she had been meeting all the usual developmental landmarks. She had finished high school, but not wished to attend university. She had been very involved in many sports, and described herself as having been pretty much a tomboy during her adolescence. She loved animals and had owned horses from her childhood, and thus was pleased with the job she had found for herself at a veterinary hospital. She came from a well-to-do family and her parents were very supportive of her. She had an older brother who owned a business in another city.

Mrs Innes's job was terminated by her employer because she could no longer handle the work she had been hired to do. She became very distraught, her pain worsened, and she was referred to the pain clinic with a recommendation that she be given psychological support.

When she presented at the pain clinic, her level of distress was very obvious. She simply could not believe that her whole life could have been so easily turned upside down in but a matter of weeks. Regarding her psychological state, her denial had just collapsed about the implications of her rheumatoid arthritis. Now she had to confront reality and come to terms with a potentially very debilitating disease. Mrs Innes's assumptive world had vanished. She cried through most of the early sessions of psychotherapy, unable to say very much. With time, however, she began to express her fears and disappointments. She became obsessed by her disease and totally preoccupied with issues of her mobility, giving elaborate accounts of each and every one of her joints that had so far been affected.

This period lasted some two months. Then her disease became quiescent. She was responding well to treatment, and there was some diminution in her preoccupation with health matters. Very tentatively she began to consider her future, while continuing to actively test the limits of her physical capacity. For instance, she embarked on the ambitious project of painting her house. When she discovered that she had taken on what was beyond her physical capabilities, in fact, she regressed and become angry, despairing, and self-deprecating.

This kind of testing went on for some months, before Mrs Innes began to show some appreciation of her physical limitations. A major turning point in the course of her psychotherapeutic treatment was her announcement to the therapist that she was planning to spend a few hours a week as a volunteer at a local daycare centre. At about this time, her husband had decided to go into business for himself. Unexpectedly, this opened up some new opportunities for Mrs Innes. Her husband is a remarkable person: supportive, understanding, and generally very optimistic about life, taking his wife's illness in his stride, providing help and encouragement. He became a major support in enabling her courage in confronting her illness and achieving some mastery over it. It can be argued that he played an important role in Mrs Innes's struggle in coming to terms with her losses and the grief that followed. Through all of this, Mrs Innes was beginning to redefine herself. When she lost her job, she fell into believing that the only identity left available to her was that of a disabled person. In seeing herself so, all her grief became tied to her lost possibilities and lost dreams.

Through psychotherapy, together with the support of her husband, her parents, and her brother, as well as her own determination, a slow process of redefining who and what she was set in. Gradually, Mrs Innes began to involve herself in her husband's business, initially making appointments and helping out with the office work. Then she took some computer courses in accounting, and before much longer took over the business side of the enterprise. Mrs Innes was discharged after eighteen months of psychotherapy with the clear understanding that she could return at any time. That was three years ago.

Analysis

Mrs Innes's story is one of loss and grief, but also one of hope. Chronic illness often requires some redefinition of identity, and most identity problems in chronic illness revolve around loss. By the time she finished psychotherapy, Mrs Innes was well on her way in coming to terms with living with the uncertainty course and consequences of a progressive chronic disease, and her altered circumstances. Was her grieving process analogous to that of someone in reaction to the death of a loved one or to a major physical loss such as loss of a limb? The differences are telling. There was no obvious or permanent loss. Even the loss of her job, while an assault on her self-esteem represented nothing like a permanent state of unemployment. In jeopardy was her health. The course of her illness was unpredictable and this was at the core of her anxiety.

Charmaz (1999) made the point that for many chronically sick people, adverse events occur sporadically from time to time, their occurrences separated by long periods of disease inactivity. Uncertainty as to what the next adverse event was going to be, and when it would occur contributed to the dread that had overtaken Mrs Innes's state of mind. The course and consequences of many if not most chronic disorders are unpredictable. Together with the primary symptoms of the illness, uncertainty about what the future thereby implies can be overwhelming for the patient. Nevertheless, Mrs Innes's health and functioning improved considerably during the eighteen months that she was in psychotherapy. Clearly, she went through a discernible period of mourning. She mourned the loss of her job, which was directly related to the loss of her health, and in doing so began the process of coming to terms with the reality of having to live with a painful, debilitating, and unpredictable disease for the rest of her life.

Abraido-Lanza (1997) studied 109 Latina women with arthritis. He reported that their important role identities contributed to the feelings of competence, such as self-esteem and self-efficacy, experienced by these women which in turn contributed to their psychological well-being. He also noted, and this is critical, that competence mediated the effects of pain, wounded identity, and illness overall. Chronic illness was found to be most devastating when it interfered with what the individual perceived as her important roles in life. The loss of roles perceived to be unimportant, however, had no such adverse effect on psychological well-being. In the case of young Mrs Innes, we might bear in mind that losing her job because of arthritis thoroughly compromised her self-esteem and her sense of self-efficacy. Her other role, that of wife, was as yet in the formative stages and seemed to be severely thrown off course by her illness. It is during the first few years of their marriage that couples establish rules and roles. That process of negotiations between two partners had apparently been brought to a halt since her illness became active. It is, therefore, not surprising that Mrs Innes's psychological health suffered a serious setback.

On the basis of the evidence to date, however, it is reasonable to be optimistic about Mrs Innes's future. The key question is what enabled Mrs Innes to redefine herself, and in doing so forsake her old dreams and find meaning and satisfaction in new roles that she slowly undertook to carve out for herself. She was fortunate in having a particularly solid social support network. She was young and intelligent, and during this time her disease did reach a fairly quiescent state. Nevertheless, she did overcome the following problems: First, and foremost, she became able to confront her own potentially debilitating disease. Second, she became able to accept the loss of some of her physical abilities, which she had valued greatly, and find meaningful alternatives. Third, she learned to accept on a day-to-day basis the vagaries of an uncertain disease. Fourth, and perhaps the most challenging, she became able to redefine her identity and to appreciate that some things had not changed even though she had a chronic illness. She was still her husband's wife. What did change was the nature of their marriage relationship. Furthermore, Mrs Innes was still a daughter and a sister. The reciprocal nature of these relationships was drastically altered, leaving her feeling less than equal. This was in addition to the task of accepting her less than perfect body, her ongoing preoccupation with her disease and a search for some meaning in her misfortune.

Leventhal and associates investigated the impact of chronic illness on the self. They observed that 'a striking aspect of disabling illness is the ability to focus attention on physical activities and bodily functions previously taken for granted' (1999: 195). Mrs Innes's preoccupation with her body bordered on obsessiveness. Month to month she was preoccupied with the anticipation of what her blood tests might reveal. If the tests showed a rise in disease activity, but subjectively she was feeling well, this apparent lack of congruency would leave her feeling distraught. She became hypervigilant of every joint in her body, and would make careful note of any hint of discomfort in any, thus far, uninvolved joint. In this way she started to reformulate herself. Through this process, she developed a realistic appreciation of the limits of her body and extricated herself from her pattern of overdoing things (counterphobic activities), which is common in the early stages of illness, just to 'prove' that she was all right.

Mrs Innes's acceptance of her medical condition came to be expressed in positive ways. She devised what Leventhal et al. (1999) described as self-defining tasks, especially of her pre-illness self. For Mrs Innes these self-defining tasks involved all her physical abilities, whether working with animals or riding her horse or participating in athletic activities. She also had to realign her newly acquired role as wife, which involved both drastic readjustments and altered expectations. In short, the core of parts of Mrs Innes's self-definition were put at serious risk by her illness. The non–self-defining tasks were also disrupted, and these mainly involved routine chores. Her true self-defining tasks were rooted in her love for animals, her physical skills, and her interpersonal relationships. Her inability to maintain her customary level of success at these tasks led to almost overwhelming grief which eventually brought her into psychotherapy. However, Mrs Innes's strength lay in her ability to change her self-defining tasks. Simply put, the transformation was from her love of physical work to more cerebral pursuits. Her personal relationships regained some of the essential elements of reciprocity, while taking into account the variability in her day-to-day pain and energy levels. She could feel that her sense of autonomy was being restored. Mrs Innes is a success story. Unfortunately, as some of the cases discussed below will show, the process of redefining oneself in the face of a chronic disorder is filled with hazards and failure and not always as successful. For many people, grieving their lost identity becomes a daily and relentless struggle. Before looking at more cases that illustrate the many facets of a patient's struggle with identity, we will briefly consider some of the literature on chronic illness and identity.

LITERATURE REVIEW

People derive a sense of what and who they are on the basis of their perceived roles. Some of these roles are pre-determined, and some acquired, such as one's partner-relationship or occupation. Gender and roles are inextricably related, even though some of the historical rigidities are undergoing major if not revolutionary changes. Whose children or siblings we are is something over which we have no control. Nevertheless, roles are inherent in all these identities and relationships.

A major role for an adult in our society is that of a worker. The significance and centrality of this role might explain the importance attached to the successful performance of it. Our work enables us not only to meet the financial obligations vital to our livelihood. Our role as worker is one that is universally valued in our society. Work defines our position in the family, society, and the social world we inhabit. In the context of chronic illness, the loss of the role of worker, as examined in the previous chapter, is tantamount to capital punishment. Loss of their role as worker for many patients with a chronic disorder is confirmation that their status as being chronically sick and disabled is irrevocable, while their status of being a viable, normal human being is severely compromised.

Chronic illness gives its sufferer a new identity, or at least changes the weighting of various attributes characteristic of the pre-illness identity. According to Charmaz (1999) the following are some key points relevant in this regard. (1) Most identity problems revolve around loss. This was evident in the case of Mrs Innes's whose problems, as we saw, emanated from her inability to perform her tasks. (2) Losses in chronic illness affect men and women differently. This is mainly a product of the differential roles and obligations that men and women continue to have in our society. The same chronic illness is likely to have different consequences for a mother with a young child than for the father of that young child should he be the principal or only breadwinner, and yet different consequences if the mother is a single parent and sole breadwinner. (3) Loss of a part of one's body or one's bodily functions, whether visible or invisible to others affects one's identity. Patients with chronic pain problems often complain that because their condition is invisible, many people including healthcare professionals do not take their suffering seriously. Some even question the existence of their condition and suggest malingering, instead, contributing loss of credibility to the patient's already lost health. This leads to shame, anger, alienation, depression and any number of other possible adverse reactions. Visible losses, such as any kind of disfigurement, also give rise to shame and make the process of coming to terms with the loss a greater struggle. (4) Chronically sick people may lose a clear sense of inner and outer boundaries. Often their pre-morbid world shrinks, and a great deal of both their inner life and their external activities revolve around the illness. (5) Being singled out and stigmatized dramatizes the differences between such patients and others and magnifies their loss. This particular issue is currently being discussed in relation to HIV patients and their struggle with their identity.

For the chronically sick, then, redefining identity in terms of their illness is a key issue. Confirmation of this critically important fact was made by Bartos and McDonald (2000), who studied seventy-six people in Australia who were living with HIV/AIDS. They found that taking HIV as their new identity was most characteristic of gay men upon learning of their diagnosis, resulting in failure to comply with treatment and/or failure to practise safe sex. Here the implication is that where the disease itself becomes integral to the new identity, the separation between the 'sickness' and 'well-being' is likely to become blurred. Nord (1997) reported that an individual's sense of self can be transformed through identification with the disease. He noted that in the gay community, a strong identification with AIDS was evident. This has led to a tendency to assume an identity based on relationship to HIV such as 'I am HIV positive [negative].' Nord observed that frequently it appeared that HIV survivors' interpersonal connections with the world, especially their connections with a community, became severely shaken. Brauhn (1999), however, reported that with the introduction of new drugs, HIV/AIDS seems increasingly to be experienced as a chronic illness, albeit with an uncertain trajectory that profoundly and pervasively affects the identity of people who have it. Lewis (1999) described how the process of accommodation to HIV and to the associated social stigma and compromised identity are different from what patients with most other chronic disorders have to cope with. The social stigma that accompanies HIV/AIDS places a special burden on people diagnosed with this still very much feared condition.

In a study of sixty-three individuals diagnosed as HIV-positive, Tewksbury and McGaughey (1998) showed that through a process of transformation these people developed a new identity. They named three critical events or milestones in this transformation process: testing for HIV antibodies; diagnosis and disease validation; and disclosure of HIV positively. Transformed identities were successfully acquired by those individuals who were able to accept themselves as being HIV-positive, living with HIV, and having AIDS. This investigation examined the process leading to acceptance of a disease, rather than the particular real and perceived losses that necessitated the adoption of a new identity.

Gurevich (1998) examined identity issues as experienced by thirteen HIV-positive women and found an intricate pattern of contradictions and dualities. These women would tend to assert that they were fundamentally the same people they had always been, while showing and stating that they were continually changing. The author noted that this continuity between the former and the present selves necessitated an accelerated revisitation of one's past, present, and future. These women existed in multiple, mutable, and contradictory realities that transcended temporal boundaries. In this exhaustive analysis of the thirteen women, the author was able to capture the intricacies and struggles that seem inherent to the process of redefining one's self that is triggered by learning that one has a chronic illness.

In an investigation involving twelve heterosexual HIV-positive women, Dozier (1998), observed significant differences between their coping styles and the styles of coping used by males with HIV/AIDS. Unlike HIV-positive men who desire to pass as healthy, women proudly claimed their HIV status. In contrast to males, these HIV-positive women were coping with the responsibilities of child care, their feelings of guilt over leaving their children in other people's care, and the adaptations accompanying being cared for rather than being the caregiver. Implicit in this study is the notion that women who are HIV-positive tend to differ from HIV-positive men in their experience of the hazards encountered in coping with the infection, especially if they have dependent children and are thus used to being in the role of caregivers.

This very brief incursion into the recent HIV and identity literature confirms the results of previous studies depicting the

struggle around coming to terms with this still dreaded condition. In addition, however, a segment of the population that is
both HIV-positive and gay seems to adopt HIV as an integral
part of their self-identity. They seem to be saying that being
HIV-positive is an attribute of identity no different from that of
being a teacher or a male or describable by any other noun one
might choose in defining ourselves. This is a new insight into
understanding and explaining the process and the tools employed in the changing self-identity and/or self-definition made
necessary by chronic illness. The gender issues are of great
clinical import. As HIV/AIDS by its uncertain course begins to
resemble any other chronic disease, we may begin to be able to
generalize some of the findings from HIV/AIDS studies to people
suffering from a variety of other chronic disorders. Nevertheless, HIV/AIDS continues to carry horrendous social stigma
which makes the question of identity and self-definition for
these patients far more troublesome and complex. The next
case we discuss involves a man who in his early forties developed a chronic pain condition that left him with no other role
or identity than that of being chronically sick.

THE CHRONIC SICK ROLE: MR KELLY

Mr Kelly's history of back pain started at age twelve. When he
was in his twenties he was referred to the pain clinic for rapid
worsening of his pain. A few years later, his condition was
aggravated further by a work-related injury. He was assessed
by several orthopaedic surgeons. A CT scan revealed significant abnormalities in his spine. Suddenly he had to give up his
work as a self-employed truck driver mainly because he could
no longer do the heavy lifting required. His pain continued to
get worse and he became unresponsive to codeine. In addition,
he developed gastritis secondary to the use of narcotic medication. This patient's past medical history was unremarkable. Surgery had been suggested, which Mr Kelly had refused at the
time because it would have meant a significant loss of income
to him. There was also some concern about his suitability for
surgery, given his psychological state.

Mr Kelly grew up in a rural area. He was the younger of the two sons of very doting parents. He had quit school after Grade 9, and started working in semi-manual labourer's jobs until setting up his own business as an independent truck driver. His work record until the time of his accident was stellar. He made a very good living. At age twenty-two, he married a woman he had known all his life. There was a son by this marriage, but the marriage ended in divorce only after four or five years. Apparently, without any warning his wife had left him for another man. Mr Kelly was devastated by this unfortunate event which also coincided with his deteriorating health. He became severely depressed and made a rather serious suicidal attempt by cutting his wrist. He was found just in time by his brother and spent the next year and a half in psychiatric care. Mr Kelly was quite critical of the psychiatric treatment because it failed to restore his 'normal' life. On further probing, he was able to acknowledge that without work and without his family he felt lonely and sad much of the time. There were occasions when these feelings became overpowering and then he would visit his parents who happened to live nearby. He had access to his little son every other weekend and lived for those times. Parting with the boy on Sundays was very hard on him. Other than his parents and his brother and family, Mr Kelly had no friends and no social life. He spent a lot of time just sitting around.

Analysis

This man went from leading a full life with his wife and a child, while being self-employed, to enduring a high level of disability. This is a perilous fall. Everything Mr Kelly valued and that gave meaning to his life, being a partner, a parent, and a self-employed worker, was lost to him within a very short space of time. Suicide must have appealed to him as the only way of ending his suffering. He was left with the chronically sick patient as the principle attribute of his identity. The magnitude of the change in Mr Kelly's self-definition and identity was almost beyond exaggeration. What does it mean to have as one's central identity the label 'chronically ill patient'? To answer that question, we have to make a brief incursion into the interrelated concepts of sick role and chronically sick role.

The sociological literature frequently addresses these two concepts. Parsons suggested that the sick role comprises two rights and two duties. A person who is sick has (1) a right to be exempt from normal social roles and (2) a right not to be held responsible for the condition. The sick person also has (3) a duty to try and get well and (4) a duty to seek and cooperate with technically competent help. Parsons's conceptualization has come under sustained criticism over the years, as is revealed by even a brief foray into the sociological literature on this topic. From our point of view, the main criticism of the Parsonian view of the sick role is that it is limited to acute illness, and it does not at all address the complexity of the sick role in the context of chronic illness. Simply put, what are Mr Kelly's rights and obligations? He has a medical condition(s) not amenable to treatment and certainly not amenable to cure. His illness has significantly reduced any possibility of returning to his pre-morbid level of functioning.

Arluke (1988) in his critical analysis of the sick role observed that when applied to chronic illness, the sick role presented almost insurmountable problems. As an example, he noted that it may be difficult for a chronically sick individual to be exempt from everyday role responsibilities. Some patients may resist giving up certain customary roles, or it may happen that the other family members are less than willing to accept any abandonment of customary role functioning by a chronically sick member. The latter situation is not infrequently observed in the families of chronic pain patients, especially when the pain condition is idiopathic. Furthermore, the very notion of getting better for a chronically ill patient is problematic. Many chronic diseases follow idiosyncratic pathways and are progressive, and many patients continue to function at a reasonable level. It is dangerous to view chronic illness as homogeneous. Variability among patients is enormous, even for those with the same illness, for example, rheumatoid arthritis. What might be a reasonable solution to this problem?

One determinant of 'appropriate' role function is the level of disability brought on by the chronic condition. Adaptation to living with a chronic illness rather than living in expectation of a cure is obviously the optimum outcome. Even this rather elastic view is not without its problems. Who and what determines, for example, if Mr Kelly is functioning at an appropriate level and has adapted well? In fact, divergence in medical opinions combined with the patient's own perception of functional capacity is at the heart of many of the conflicts between workers compensation boards, employers, insurance companies, and patients (Roy 2001). In short, assuming the chronic sick role is fraught with difficulties and conflicts both for the patient and for society at large.

The chronic sick role fell upon Mr Kelly, and when combined with the failure of his marriage, had far-reaching consequences. Let us briefly consider the remaining roles open to Mr Kelly. He is still a very engaged, part-time parent; and he continues to be a son to his parents, although the quality of this relationship has undergone major changes. Mr Kelly's parents now are his almost only source of social support. Mr Kelly continues to carry out some of his essential role functions such as taking care of himself. Charmaz (1999) noted that sick people relinquish some identities, while retaining others. Nevertheless, it was obvious to any observer that Mr Kelly had relinquished most of his valued identities, leaving him with a very damaged sense of who and what he is. Even as a father to his young son, Mr Kelly feels both his physical as well as financial limitations. His wife left him for another man, which would seriously challenge any husband's core identity as a man. Mr Kelly has little doubt that he has been deprived of everything that he finds important.

Why is this story so different from that of Mrs Innes, who also developed a very serious and challenging medical condition? It is hard to overlook that while Mrs Innes's story was one of cautious optimism, Mr Kelly's situation offers few grounds for hope.

One obvious difference is their respective medical conditions. Mrs Innes had rheumatoid arthritis, whereas Mr Kelly is in chronic pain triggered by trauma. Both situations are filled with uncertainty, but with one distinction. Mrs Innes's rheumatoid arthritis emerged over a considerable period of time, and although she was long in denial, the disease continued to progress. Yet, she at least had the opportunity to reflect on the vicissitudes of living with rheumatoid arthritis. For Mr Kelly the debilitation was sudden and entirely unanticipated. His life was turned upside down in a flash. In the early stages of his disabled condition, there was enormous uncertainty regarding his prognosis. This leads to a second observation. While Mrs Innes's symptoms improved with treatment, Mr Kelly's continued to deteriorate with the net result that he lost his trucking business – thus his job and livelihood.

Third, and this is critical, these two individuals experienced different life events. Mrs Innes lost her job, which signalled the beginning of her struggle. Mr Kelly not only lost his job, but at about the same time his wife left him, taking their young son with her. In short, concurrently Mr Kelly was confronted with several enormous negative events, both related and unrelated to his medical condition, which left him psychologically far more vulnerable than Mrs Innes ever was. Mr Kelly became clinically depressed and required prolonged treatment. Mrs Innes, whose principle problem was reactive grief, was able to recover her sense of well-being with psychotherapy alone.

Fourth, Mrs Innes was fortunate in a number of ways. She came from a wealthy family with very strong attachments to both her parents and a sibling. She had a very caring husband. She was part of a network of friends and continued to have an active social life. In contrast, Mr Kelly, also with supportive parents, had to contend with the humiliation of being left by his wife for another man and together with that humiliation, losing his son (except for visits). Mr Kelly's assumptive world simply collapsed, and his social support system was inadequate in serving as any kind of buffer for his suffering. The contrast between these two individuals is most striking in terms of social support.

Fifth, Mr Kelly, being rapidly faced with health and marital problems, rapidly decompensated. Mrs Innes, even in the early stages of psychotherapy, showed signs of redirecting her talents and energy. For example, Mrs Innes started volunteering at a daycare centre. Circumstances pulled these two people in exactly opposite directions. While Mrs Innes searched for new identities, Mr Kelly sank ever deeper into the chronic sick role and disability.

Mrs Innes, although fearful of her illness, was able to maintain some of her central identity roles. She was determined not to succumb to her illness. Her greatest fear lay in the uncertainties of her disease. At first, she coped by overactivity, which was part of her denial mechanism. Nevertheless, Mrs Innes was not willing to accept seeing herself as limited to being a disabled and chronically sick person. In contrast, Mr Kelly was overwhelmed by having lost at once everything that he valued: his job, his wife, and his child, as well as his health. Confronted with these losses, not only was Mr Kelly unable to maintain at least some of critical elements of his identity, but he basically lost all sense of who and what he was, which culminated in a serious attempt at suicide.

Finally, the availability of opportunities for these two individuals was worlds apart. Mrs Innes, in relatively short time regained her self-esteem by working as a partner in her husband's business. As already noted, she discovered her talents for running the day-to-day affairs of the business in addition to deliberately acquiring computer skills. Even after making considerable progress in recovering from his depression, Mr Kelly had no such opportunities readily available to him. It is conceivable that Mr Kelly might have been able to engage in some meaningful activities, in spite of his pain, had the opportunity for doing so presented itself. Such was not the case. As the level of motivation to take charge of her life increased in Mrs Innes, sadly, the opposite was true with Mr Kelly.

CONCLUSION

The two cases discussed in this chapter reveal the difficulties inherent in making any sweeping generalizations about the impact of chronic illness on identity. Recently, a man in his early seventies presented at our clinic with a history of severe irritable bowel syndrome. In the very first interview, it was obvious that this was a very disabled person whose daily life was dominated by pain and suffering. In due course, however, it emerged that he and his wife went to restaurants several times a week; during summer months they went on car rides once or twice a week, and they regularly visited with friends. In addition, this patient regularly spent quite a bit of time tending his flowers.

What might account for this man's apparently over-reaction in viewing himself as disabled? To some extent an answer might be revealed by his history. This man's pain conditions (he also suffers from idiopathic back pain), although of many years' duration, became significantly worse soon after he retired. He had taken early retirement from his railroad conductor's job so that he could spend more time with his wife. His disappointment in reaction to his deteriorating health was at the root of his exaggerated sense of disability. When these facts emerged, this patient was asked directly whether he viewed himself as sick or disabled. At first it was very difficult to elicit a direct response from him. However, when challenged by being told that he seemed to be living a rather full life, he acknowledged that one of his dreams had been to travel after retirement, and now he had become a little fearful of doing so. The point of this man's story is that self-definition following loss and disability is not infrequently at odds with reality. This patient was far from disabled. Although his view of himself was associated to a large degree with what he believed would remain his unfulfilled dreams; objectively, he was not disabled.

This man's case, along with the other two cases discussed in this chapter point to a critical problem in determining the extent of the loss of identity. One person redefined her priorities and almost created a new sense of self; while another patient was left with almost no identity other than that of a disabled individual, and as another variant, our last patient had thoroughly overestimated the loss resulting from his illness. In the midst of these varied and complex situations, issues of uncertainty about the course of the illness, personal attributes that determine individual response, and the severity of the medical condition further complicate the picture.

Uncertainty, although commonly experienced by chronically ill and/or disabled patients, has many faces. First and foremost, one must consider whether the disease is amenable to treatment, as was the case with Mrs Innes. Frequently, with many untreatable chronic conditions, uncertainty comes from not being able to predict the course that the disease might follow. Uncertainty is present also with treatable conditions, where the fear is one of relapse or rapid deterioration in the future. With many conditions even day-to-day variations in the patient's sense of well-being become a major source of anxiety. These variations are not always readily explainable, but can be based on the patient's subjective feelings. Another kind of uncertainty is reported by people suffering from painful and debilitating conditions that are episodic. Migraine falls into that category. Patients have reported living with a certain amount of foreboding about a migraine attack which, in spite of significant improvements in treatment, can severely disrupt life for short periods of time.

It is obvious that threat to identity as a result of chronic illness is unpredictable. For these patients the loss of their important roles in life has far-reaching consequences. Precisely what factors determine the response to loss of roles and therefore one's self-definition must be regarded as somewhat unpredictable. Unquestionably, the degree of disability is a key factor. Even here there is a great deal of variability. It does happen that very disabled individuals can show remarkable resilience and in the face of seemingly insurmountable odds lead fulfilling lives.

Any discussion of roles necessarily leads to an exploration of the sociological underpinnings of role as a concept. Sociological perspectives, however, have to be integrated into the clinical. The central clinical issue here in respect to loss of identity as a result of chronic illness and disability is the struggle our patients have to work out this loss. The task they face is the discovery of new meanings in whatever sense of self they are left with. Let us consider an illustration of this. A man with severe herpes zoster was very incapacitated by this painful disorder. He was almost totally confined to his house, and the family took on caring for all of his needs. Sometimes, this man would express a desire to make a cup of coffee for his wife now and then, or to go out to the local store to get a newspaper, or perhaps just dust the furniture. He wanted to feel useful within the limits of his disabilities.

Redefining oneself when much is lost through chronic illness is at best an overwhelming task. Partly this is because it is also, to some extent, a moving target. Charmaz (1999) proposed three critical steps for the chronically ill in relation to the struggle that accompanies preservation of identity. They are: (1) recapturing the past; (2) preserving a public identity and changing a private one; and (3) developing strategies for preserving the self. As a conclusion to this chapter, we shall briefly discuss our two patients, Mrs Innes and Mr Kelly, in the context of these three steps.

The effort to recapture the past, or more precisely, avoiding the danger of losing even more of one's identity, left Mrs Innes in a prolonged period of denial. The deterioration in health was slow but steady, until she reached a point where it became impossible for her to function. Her profound sadness upon losing her job was at the heart of her inability to maintain her most valued sense of self, and only after working through her grief and coming to terms with her illness was she able to reshape her identity as a productive and vibrant human being once again.

Mr Kelly, on the other hand, lost his wife and health suddenly without warning, and both almost at the same time. The assault of these events on his self was profound. His past had been taken away from him and he held little hope of regaining it. Mr Kelly clung to the remnants of his past valiantly, mainly through being a very part-time father to his young son. He was not as fortunate as Mrs Innes. To begin the process of redefining himself in any positive way, Mr Kelly had very little left of his past sources of support and self-esteem.

Charmaz (1999) noted that some men try to retain their public identities in reaffirming their past and demonstrate continuity into the present. Mrs Innes made a conscious effort in this direction. She continued to work as a veterinarian's assistant despite her pain and sense of foreboding. However, all her efforts to maintain her previous public identity came to a dramatic end when her employment was abruptly terminated. There was no longer any way of minimizing the effects of her rheumatoid arthritis.

All of Mr Kelly's public identities were dramatically removed. Not only was he not able to remain connected with his public identities, but in fact, they were transformed. From being a self-employed, married man with a child, he became a psychiatric in-patient following his suicide attempt ensuing from his new status as a chronic pain patient that followed upon his accident. There was no way for Mr Kelly to preserve any public identity.

Finally, let us examine the strategies patients employ to preserve a sense of self and some continuity. In this respect, Mrs Innes's story is instructive and optimistic. Despite her rather short-term upheaval, she was very fortunate in many respects. She herself was very determined to reshape her life, and she was blessed with a very strong and effective social support network. In addition, her disease retreated. She was able to develop a strategy for redefining who and what she is, and she has been very successful in achieving the new goals she set for herself. Mr Kelly, for all the facts that we know about him, was simply devoid of any strategies. He became excessively dependent on his parents again, and in many ways regressed into the position of a young and dependent child. His parents were only too pleased to help him in any way they could.

These two individuals give us some indication of the critical social, psychological, and medical factors that can begin to explain how two very different trajectories of the struggle with identity following loss can lead to two very different outcomes.

5

Family Roles: What Is Lost?

This is a continuation of the preceding chapter. Here we are concerned specifically with the loss of family roles. These losses present a serious challenge to chronic patients' sense of self. We have so far examined loss of work, as well as the implications of both the sick role and the chronically sick role. The family roles are so critical because of their multifaceted nature. As has already been emphasized, we all derive our sense of who and what we are from the performance of our various roles. The significance of our role in our family probably outweighs any other of our roles. Most of us consider our family to be the most important component of their lives.

Tunks and Roy (1982) noted that human roles are those behavioural programs which are carried out by individuals according to societal expectations and rules, they are stable over time, allow for predictability and are compatible with the rules governing others in the environment, and the roles are complementary to the roles of others within that ecological system. Roles serve the purpose of maintaining social order by reducing dissonance or distress, allowing for adaptation, and providing a basis for satisfaction. This is a comprehensive interpretation of roles that takes into account a number of critical variables. In the case of a person becoming chronically ill, and possibly no longer be able to fulfil hitherto expected roles, the new situation has implications for both that person and the ecological system in which that person is located. We have considered some of the trials and tribulations of change in the identity of patients faced with chronic illness or disability. Changes in family roles have far-reaching psychological effects on them and are often a major source of family discord.

Family roles are complex, yet the literature on the loss of these roles for the chronically sick is rather limited. Many aspects of family life in relation to arthritic disorders, which are widely prevalent in the population, have been examined in the literature and may offer a reasonable prototype for chronic disorders (Danoff-Burg and Revenson, 2000; Dowdy, 1999; Poole, 2000; Reisine, 1995; Reisine and Fifield, 1995; Whitley-Reed, 1999). However, no study has reported on the aspect of losing one's family roles. In a recent paper, Barlow et al. (1999) did examine the emotional responses of arthritic patients to their failure in being able to fulfil their expected roles. These patients' perceived inability to fulfil their roles, especially as parents with young children, resulted in feelings of frustration, guilt, anger, and even depression. Reisine (1995), in a review of the literature on arthritis and family, noted that much of it centred on family functioning and, by inference, not on patients' response to the loss of their roles. Roy (1989), in his analyses of 32 families of whom thirteen patients suffered from chronic low back pain and nineteen with chronic headache, found role dysfunction to be pervasive. Even provision of resources, a basic family task, had been seriously compromised for several of the back pain families. The family breadwinners had lost their jobs, and the families now found themselves in dire financial circumstances. This illustrates how roles are intertwined. We can add that the majority of the families of chronically ill patients are less than adequate in performing their affective roles, especially in the area of nurturance and support.

Family therapy researchers have developed tools with which to explore family roles. There is universal recognition of the pivotal significance of overall family functioning. Dysfunction in family roles is often at the root of family problems. Consider a mother of two young children who periodically becomes unable to function for several days at a time when she in the throes of a migraine headache. If there is adequate family support, and others are available to take over the slack created by this mother's temporary illness, the family may continue to function reasonably well. If such support is unavailable, however, the family is put at some risk. If the condition is more debilitating, even permanent, then the issues confronting a family become very serious, indeed.

In this chapter we will explore a variety of responses to the loss of valued family roles by our patients upon becoming chronically sick or disabled. For the purpose of analyses we shall use the role component of the McMaster Model Family Functioning (MMFF) which to date remains the most comprehensive such model. Several research instruments for family assessment are based on the MMFF, including the Family Assessment Device (FAD) and the Family Assessment Measure (FAM). Roles according to the McMaster model include instrumental and affective roles. Instrumental roles consist of functions that relate to the provision of resources, life-skills development, and the management and maintenance of the family system. Affective roles involve nurturing and support and sexual gratification for sexual partners, which is the topic of the next chapter. The literature on the negative effects of chronic illness on family functioning is replete with methodological concerns, some of them serious (Roy, 2001). Nevertheless, little doubt exists that many families are adversely affected when one of their members develops a chronic illness. In contrast to the literature on job loss and its psychological fallout, the literature has so far paid little attention to individual responses to the loss of family roles. But even though psychological reactions to the role changes brought on by chronic illness are under-researched, there is general consensus that at the very least loss of roles and changes in family roles and rules about who does what is very stressful to all concerned. Here we shall examine a number of cases regarding the nature, extent, and consequences of the loss of family-related roles in relation to patients with chronic illness.

A CASE OF GREAT FAMILY DISRUPTION: MRS LYNN

Mrs Lynn had a prolonged history of headache which suddenly left her health so deteriorated that she had to quit her job. Thereupon, she became very distressed. Mrs Lynn was married, and had two children, John, aged nineteen, and Ann, aged twelve. Prior to the onset of her severe headaches, she had been a caring mother and partner engaged in all family activities, taking immense pride and satisfaction in her relationship with her husband and children.

This stable family situation was severely tested when Mrs Lynn's headaches worsened to the point that she became so disabled she could not work. She also became clinically depressed. The depression was immediately diagnosed, and she was placed on antidepressant medication. Unfortunately, Mrs Lynn did not respond well to this pharmacological treatment. Meanwhile, her family situation worsened. She became totally disengaged from her roles and functions as a mother and spouse. Mrs Lynn began to spend large amounts of time in her bedroom, refusing to see anyone. She cried a great deal, and for days on end would refuse to eat. Her daughter's behaviour took a turn for the worse.

The rest of the family learned to fend for themselves. While babysitting, Ann stole some entirely useless articles from their neighbour. She made no effort to conceal her crime, and was easily found out by her father. He did not make a big issue of it, but when Mrs Lynn found out, she became very angry and severely chastised Ann. In addition, John became very aloof, and would spend all the daylight hours away from home. Increasingly, Ann became defiant, while correspondingly, her mother became inconsistent in her behaviour towards Ann, and also towards her husband. Mr Lynn was beginning to show signs of frustration at the lack of apparent progress in his wife's condition, which he expressed mainly by silence (passive-aggressive behaviour). He remained very sympathetic to Ann. Mrs Lynn's conditions, migraine and depression, remained impervious to treatment, and although she experienced brief periods of relief from pain and depression, both appeared to be chronic. Let us examine Mrs Lynn's family roles applying the McMaster Model.

Provision of Resources

Mrs Lynn had been very much the 'manager' of the household. She ensured that essential tasks like purchasing food and paying bills were carried out, and in this respect Mr Lynn had played only a marginal role. But then drastic changes occurred in Mrs Lynn's activities. Much of her former family responsibility fell on Mr Lynn, who became resentful of this change. Mrs Lynn, in her turn, was never to be quite satisfied with her husband's new efforts and openly critical of what she called his lack of 'common sense.' Mrs Lynn experienced much frustration, as well as guilt, over her inability to consistently perform her usual tasks, and her only 'strength' was to express disaffection with her husband's performance. Yet, the basic tasks of buying grocery, paying bills, and preparing meals, were being accomplished quite adequately by Mr Lynn, with the help of the children.

Life-Skills Development

The role of household manager includes functions that affect both the children and the adults in the family. Various efforts are necessary in helping children commence and complete school, in helping an adult pursue a career or vocational interest, and in maintaining or improving each family member's level of personal development. These constitute the tasks necessary for life-skills development.

The Lynn family suffered serious set-backs in role functioning. Mrs Lynn had been very devoted in her involvement with her children's education and day-to-day activities. She wanted them to grow up as healthy, happy, and responsible citizens. Mrs Lynn had taken considerable pride in the children's scholastic achievements, was the main source of support for her husband, who held a responsible position at work. Then she began to withdraw almost totally from these tasks. And unlike the tasks associated with his role as family breadwinner, Mr Lynn was not able to fill the gap left by the changes in his wife. This gave him feelings of inadequacy. Mrs Lynn's helplessness and frustration were significantly aggravated when she learned that her daughter Ann was being truant from school, and generally otherwise engaging in unacceptable behaviours. Mrs Lynn responded to these situations with anger which, predictably, only aggravated the situation further. In therapy, Mrs Lynn talked about how her whole world was slipping away from her, and how she felt utterly helpless to do anything to stop this. She retreated from the world even further. Apparently, her son John seemed to remain unaffected by all the turbulence in the family.

Maintenance and Management of the System

The family aspect of role function addresses questions such as who is involved in major decision making, with whom does the final decision rest, who settles family disputes, who monitors children's health, or who determines decisions such as going to the doctor or seeking advice outside the family when needed? Mrs Lynn was substantially in all these activities, as well as others. Her withdrawal from them left the family with huge enormous problems which no one else was able to solve. She undoubtedly had been the key decision maker in the family, and the underlying reason for this arrangement was that Mr Lynn worked very long hours and was quite simply not around. Mrs Lynn, as a result of her chronic pain condition and depression, could do nothing but watch as the family seemed to fall apart around her.

Nurturance and Support

Nurturance and support are primarily affective roles. The associated tasks lead family members to provide each other love, reassurance, support, understanding, affection, care, and comfort. Not only was Mrs Lynn unable to fulfil these functions, much as she did want to, in a curious way, she found herself being less wanted and less needed. Other than her son, both her husband and the daughter became somewhat hostile to her, and all of the positive emotions in this family soured. Mrs Lynn responded to her dismay by further excluding herself from emotional involvement, and occasionally she emerged only to heap criticism on her daughter and husband. Ann felt almost totally abandoned, and her antisocial activities were becoming potentially criminal. Furthermore, there are the roles of adult sexual gratification and marital or spousal roles which form the topic for the next chapter.

Analysis

This account of the loss of family roles for Mrs Lynn does not begin to reflect the enormity of the upheaval her illness caused the family or the inner turmoil it caused her. The active phase of Mrs Lynn's illness lasted about three years. The variety of family complications associated with depression in a mother is described in the literature (Roy, 2001; see Chapter 4). Chronic pain and depression have been reported to coexist in a high proportion of chronic pain patients (Thomas and Roy, 1999; see Chapter 6). Our patients, like Mrs Lynn, frequently find themselves in a situation of double jeopardy. The chronic pain condition in a family member is alone capable of disrupting family roles, but when combined with clinical depression, the consequences are often more far reaching. Despite her condition, Mrs Lynn was at all times aware of the chaos her illness had brought on her family. Her feelings of guilt and shame only exacerbated her depression.

It must be obvious that Mrs Lynn was caught in a difficult cycle. She was full of dismay and guilt in reaction to her failure to fulfil the tasks involved with her accustomed roles. These feelings were further exacerbated by her realization that her inability to function was a major cause of the great disharmony that had overtaken her family. The whole spectrum of family roles became compromised for Mrs Lynn.

The gender of the patient and the life stage of the family are two issues that merit attention here. That Mrs Lynn was disabled as a mother and a wife produced particular reaction in the other family members as well as in herself. Unlike perhaps some other families, Mrs Lynn was clearly the manager as well as the principal caretaker of this family. She provided balance and equanimity for all family members. Her husband relied on her not only for the management of the household, but also for being the link with the outside world and the primary source of emotional support for himself and the children.

Evidence supports the contention that illness in a mother affects the family quite differently from when the patient is the father (Roy, 2001; see Chapter 4). In his analysis of thirty-two families where one member had chronic pain Roy (1989) found that women headache patients, whether full-time workers or homemakers or both, carried major responsibilities for care of the children and household chores. Mothers even today are more involved in child-rearing, providing emotional support, love, and nurturance, while doing a much greater share of the housework, than are the fathers. For all of these reasons, when a mother is removed from performing some or all of these roles through illness or disability, her family experiences a major upheaval. Such upheaval, in turn, puts additional emotional distress on the mother, who is already not well.

The impact on the mother on seeing her own inability to perform these tasks can be devastating. A seriously disabled patient in our clinic, who also had a chronic pain condition, said that she could see her family become unglued, and there was very little she could do about it. If she had been sad and despondent before this, watching her family as it fell apart had made her desperate. Women patients, unlike their male partners, try very hard to maintain their nurturing as well as family maintenance roles. This was clearly so in Mrs Lynn's case. Her illness removed the factor that had kept this family in a state of some stability. Mr Lynn was singularly unable to fill the vacuum left by his wife's involuntary abandonment of her role functions. Indeed, he found himself puzzled by her 'wilful' behaviour, and at times wondered about whether her illness was even real.

Family Life-Stage Issues

As Thomas and Roy (1999) have reported, the patient's age at onset of the illness can have predictable repercussions for not only the patient but also the family. In Mrs Lynn's family there were two teenagers when she first became ill and incapacitated. Her son was at a point where he was showing considerable self-reliance, but her daughter Ann was at a very vulnerable age. Besides, as already noted, Mr Lynn, who was almost the same age as the patient, was very committed to his career at this time, and spent most of his waking hours at work. The daughter, in effect, 'lost' her mother at a time when she was just entering her teen years. Up to that point in time, Ann had had a close and confiding relationship with her mother. Faced with the unpredictable behaviour of her mother and an unavailable father, Ann resorted to acting-out behaviours. Mr Lynn was angry with our patient for abandoning the family, although he had a sense at some level that his anger was perhaps irrational. Still, he did not seem to possess the wherewithal to assume some of his wife's responsibilities. As will become evident with other case illustrations, the reactions of families to chronic illness affecting one of their members are determined to a significant degree by the life stage of the family and its members.

From being an effective mother, Mrs Lynn became almost completely ineffectual. From being a good mother she became 'bad,' at least in her own eyes. From being a reliant and giving spouse and partner, she became dependent on her husband, and they both, to some extent, felt failed by the other. Mrs Lynn's recovery was slow. As she gained more and more control over her pain and depression, her anger with her husband became more palpable. She felt he had betrayed her by failing to provide her with support when she so needed it, and even more importantly, by failing to keep the family together. She became single-minded in her efforts at winning her daughter back; this, too, took a couple of years. During the course of prolonged psychotherapy, Mrs Lynn gradually came to terms with her deep feelings of having been let down and of having let others down, especially, her young teenaged daughter.

Finally, it must be mentioned that Mrs Lynn, over time, did regain her central position in the family. But by that time the family had moved on to another stage. The son had left home, the daughter was soon to leave high school, and her husband no longer was quite so caught up in his job.

WHERE IS THE LOSS? — MR MORTON

Compared with Mrs Lynn's story, Mr Morton's case seems more straightforward. Mr Morton suffered from a chronic abdominal pain problem which forced him to take early retirement from his railroad job. Mr Morton was married to the same woman for more than thirty years. He married late, because he could not find the 'right' person. The marriage had been very satisfactory. When seen for the first time, for his psychosocial assessment, Mr Morton presented himself as a rather helpless individual whose life was now controlled by his ever-present pain.

Mr Morton's medical problems dated back to when he was only three or four years old. As a youngster he often had very bad leg pain. Later, from about age sixteen to twenty he had cardiac problems, involving rapid heart beat (tachycardia) intermittently, followed by periods when his heart functioned quite normally. His view of himself as long-suffering dated back to his childhood. Nevertheless, he met all his developmental landmarks. He acknowledged that he received special attention from his parents when he was ill. There was nothing extraordinary about this man's presentation and history other than an observation that being sick and receiving care and attention was very much part of his lifelong experience.

A different picture emerged during a conjoint session with his wife. Since his retirement, Mr and Mrs Morton had visited Britain together numerous times, their last such trip about two years before this. Mr Morton had enjoyed that trip, and his pain had not seemed to interfere all that much with the demands of the journey. When back at home, however, his level of functioning soon was at odds with what he had perceived it to be while away.

Here we shall make some general observations about Mr Morton's level of functioning in his family roles. In terms of necessary family functions, the couple seemed to do everything together. They shopped together. Important decisions such as purchasing a car were made together, although Mrs Morton said that she knew nothing about cars, and they managed their money together. What emerged was a picture of a harmonious relationship in which both partners played equal roles. They had a flower garden, and as Mr Morton was particularly fond of gardening, he spent a lot of time tending his flowers. Yet, Mr Morton was convinced that his abdominal disease was hindering his undertaking normal activities. This view of himself as an unwell person had deep roots. One might surmise that holding onto the view of himself as a person who was always suffering and in pain held some psychological benefit for him, mainly in the care and attention he would receive from the healthcare professionals and perhaps also his wife, who, while not minimizing his pain and discomfort, contributed greatly to the maintenance of Mr Morton's active lifestyle.

Analysis

The key question is whether Mr Morton's abdominal condition compromised his family roles? It did not appear to. Another important question here is, What are the family roles for a man in his early seventies? Necessary family functions, by definition, have to be maintained, and this couple was able to do so without difficulty. Mr Morton remained involved in his family roles to the same degree as he had prior to his illness. Although life-skills development needs are likely to be quite different for people in their seventies than for younger couples, but the nurturance and support roles remain essential. Mr Morton was in a supportive relationship characterized by mutual caring and respect, as well as the sharing of necessary tasks.

Mr and Mrs Morton were a high-functioning couple, and Mr Morton's medical condition had not compromised his family roles to any measurable degree. His wife was unable to name even one area of responsibility that Mr Morton may have abandoned because of his illness. They were quite non-traditional in their roles. He used to do all the cooking when both of them were working. Now, other than cooking, and even there he helped her in the kitchen, they shared all responsibilities. Basically, Mr Morton's medical condition had left him entirely un-impaired. That is not to deny that he had a serious abdominal condition and suffered a lot of pain.

This is an unusual case in many ways. First and foremost, Mr Morton overestimated his level of disability, and some plausible reasons for doing so have been discussed. The antecedents for this misperception of his own condition could possibly be traced back to his childhood experiences. Second, his family roles were not gender-specific, keeping in mind that this couple were never involved in child-rearing, which is a responsibility often shouldered mostly by women. Third, Mr Morton was in a supportive relationship in which there was virtually no evidence of strife. In essence, although Mr Morton very much objected to living with pain, he maintained all his meaningful family roles – almost in spite of himself. There was no loss of any family roles for Mr Morton. That reason alone makes this is somewhat of an unusual case.

WHY DOES HE NOT HELP ME? – MRS NEIL

The prolonged history of Mrs Neil's medical problems included chronic back pain due to degenerative changes, malignant melanoma, fibromyalgia, and myofascial pain syndrome. She and her husband immigrated to Canada when in their late twenties from Europe to make a new life. After struggling in menial jobs for several years, they both succeeded in obtaining employment in office management. In addition, they had both upgraded their education. They had one child, a married daughter who was a healthcare professional, and a young grandson. In spite of Mrs Neil's many health problems, she had worked for the same firm for many years. Unfortunately, especially because of her back pain, her health deteriorated to such a degree that she took early retirement.

Mrs Neil was remarkably efficient. She managed her household, raised a child, and held a responsible position – without much help from her husband. From all accounts she was happy in her marriage, and when first seen together at our clinic, they presented a history of a harmonious relationship. It was a traditional marriage, but as Mrs Neil's health deteriorated and Mr Neil showed little or no inclination to assume any household responsibilities, things became less pleasant. The entire situation spun out of control, however, when Mr Neil suffered a massive myocardial infarction which left him disabled for a long period, and forced him to retire from his demanding office manager's position.

Now they were two individuals, both impaired, both unable to carry out the routine tasks of daily living. The greater part of the burden fell on Mrs Neil, and with the help of the daughter, who also suffered from a chronic neurological problem, she somehow managed to keep the household on track. For the first time in their long marriage, Mrs Neil began to show signs of resentment towards her husband. The sources of this resentment were complicated. Signs of it began as Mrs Neil's concern for Mr Neil's singular unwillingness to participate in his treatment regime, which included regular exercise and diet control. He resisted both. However, Mrs Neil's anger took a sharper turn when she confronted him with his lack of concern not only for himself, but also for her. Housework was becoming increasingly difficult for her. Matters were made worse when Mr Neil took it upon himself to invest a considerable sum of their joint money without Mrs Neil's prior knowledge. This is when everything came to a head. After more than three decades of marriage, Mrs Neil was seriously considering divorce. They came to us seeking marriage therapy.

The division of family roles and responsibilities was at the centre of their disagreements. Mr Neil often appeared puzzled during such discussions, and generally bewildered about the purpose of the sessions they were attending at our clinic. They had always lived this way, explained Mr Neil. He was no longer working any more and his health had become compromised, but other than that everything was the same.

Analysis

Gender issues are very pronounced in this case. Mrs Neil held a full-time job outside the home and had complete responsibility for managing the household. As her health deteriorated, she tried to carry on as before, but with considerable difficulty. Mr Neil was, at best oblivious and at worst, totally callous and insensitive to Mrs Neil's burdens and difficulties. Even common sense would suggest that this husband should have been aware of his wife's considerably compromised level of functioning, and that he should have been making some effort or at least indicating a willingness to help out.

Mrs Neil's problems are frequently evident in retired couples where both partners have ongoing health problems. In the literature this topic is usually discussed under the general heading of the 'burden of caring,' and in Chapter 7 we will consider in more detail the loss of health and its consequences in the elderly. Nevertheless, in our case study here, Mrs Neil was not only confronted with fears and anxieties about her own health, but also her worries about her husband's heart attack and his response to it. The situation became altogether unbearable for her.

Mrs Neil's anger and frustration had only in part to do with the loss of family roles. It had much more to do with her husband's attitude to her difficulties and to his apparent unwillingness to take responsibility for his own health. Thus, Mrs

Neil's problems were threefold: (1) her compromised health; (2) her husband's insensitivity to her needs; and (3) her husband's indifference to his own serious health problems. This case illustrates how loss of family roles is one of many consequences of chronic illness. In this particular couple, the burden of maintaining existing family roles was complicated by an indifferent partner who was equally indifferent to his own health problems. Her partner's attitude was at the very centre of Mrs Neil's resentment, anger, and sadness. Not only, in the face of chronic pain and ill health, did she have to carry on with her usual family roles, but now she had to assume responsibility for her husband's well-being as well. It all became too much for Mrs Neil.

LOSS OF CHERISHED ROLES: MR OSCAR

Following upon a serious motor vehicle accident, Mr Oscar lost his livelihood as a businessman and much more. He was married, and the couple had three grown-up children, two of whom were still living at home. In the early stages of his disability, Mr Oscar had denied any emotional difficulties, and claimed that if only the physicians were more competent, he would have been able to go back to running his business. His hostility to the health care system was palpable. As an aside, he let it be known that he had declared business as well as personal bankruptcy.

A fuller picture of the upheaval experienced in this family as a result of Mr Oscar's disability emerged in a joint session with both Mr and Mrs Oscar. Almost all the family-related responsibilities had shifted to Mrs Oscar. For the first time in their long marriage, she suddenly had had to learn to manage the household's finances – and under very reduced circumstances – listen to the many problems that the children were having, and – also for the first time in her married life – she had had to obtain paid work outside the home. Because Mr Oscar gave very little outward sign of suffering, Mrs Oscar was unsure of what she could realistically expect from him. Nevertheless, she continued to assume all his responsibilities without a complaint.

Mrs Oscar found herself making important decisions without the benefit of his counsel. This couple's ability to work together was as much victim of a car accident as was the husband's health.

Mr Oscar was in a state of inner turmoil and confusion. He felt at odds with himself, particularly as he withdrew from his responsibilities, but in view of being so obliged to his wife he felt that he was not permitted to express any opinion on what she was doing or contradict her in any way. He recalled how on one occasion, for example, he had tried to carry some shopping bags from the car to the house, but his wife had stopped him. As Mrs Oscar took on more and more responsibilities, Mr Oscar was left with virtually no right to an opinion. He felt hopeless and helpless. In therapy he was able to express his profound sense of isolation, and his persistent thoughts of himself as a failure. There were times when he wanted to help out, but something held him back. Their children no longer came to him for advice. In happier times, he had been their soccer coach. The children's drifting away from him had been particularly hurtful. Mr Oscar used to be a successful businessman and a caring father and husband who was involved in every aspect of family life. Now, in his words, he had turned into a 'useless' person. His abrogation of family roles was almost total.

Analysis

Clearly, the Oscars used to have a well-functioning family and marriage partnership. An unexpected event – an automobile accident – had turned the family relationships, roles, and responsibilities upside-down. Role reversals were very evident. The gaps left by the patient were almost completely picked up by his wife. This did not happen without costs to the entire family. This family went from relative financial well-being to what may be termed a state of 'genteel poverty.' The role changes that occurred in the family were many and their dynamics complex. Mrs Oscar took on more and more tasks without a word and, in fact, actively discouraged Mr Oscar from doing anything lest he should hurt himself. The net effect was Mr Oscar's confusion about who and what he was.

How are we to explain Mr Oscar's behaviour? First, and foremost, we must correctly ascertain the level of his disability. Was Mr Oscar left totally disabled by the car accident? Clearly, he was not. Indeed, he actually appeared to be quite fit and able and certainly capable of doing his part in maintaining some family roles. Perhaps his withdrawal from these roles was more psychological than anything. Having lost his primary role as breadwinner, he seemed to see no purpose in doing anything else. Was he looking for a way to relinquish his family responsibilities? Did his disability provide him with a legitimate way of withdrawing from roles and responsibilities that he did not want? His past behaviour lent no support to this proposition. Mr Oscar had been engaged in every aspect of family life and had taken much pride in his roles as a father and a partner to his wife. Another possibility is that Mr Oscar was traumatized and had been depressed as a result of the suddenness as well as the magnitude of his misfortunes. This is the most likely explanation for Mr Oscar's quiet withdrawal into himself and disengagement from family life.

It is also conceivable that Mrs Oscar's behaviour was reinforcing her husband's withdrawal from the family. Certain essential tasks had to be maintained. Bills had to be paid; the family finances had been thrown into a mess, and she had to find paid employment. As Mrs Oscar assumed these responsibilities with great difficulty, her husband's self-worth suffered further setbacks, and the whole problem took on the qualities of a vicious cycle. The more that Mrs Oscar was forced to take on, or willingly took on, the more useless and hopeless her husband became. This was the state they were in when they were first presented together.

During the course of family therapy Mr Oscar, on many occasions, stated that he felt like a lodger in his own home. He felt that he had lost all his rights as a father and a husband. It hurt him enormously when he would hear his children talking to their mother in search of advice or just engaging in general chit-chat with her. The children no longer came to him. He was uncertain about the reason for this. Had he pushed them away? Or, were they avoiding him or perhaps they just did not want to bother him because of his poor health? Mr Oscar was equally perplexed by his wife's behaviour. Why wasn't she angry with him? He felt certain that she must hate him for letting her down, and so on and so forth. Self-recrimination was driving Mr Oscar's thoughts and behaviour. He believed that he had forfeited all his rights. He had no opinions on any matter, or if he did, he further believed that he had no right to express them.

As already noted, the insults to Mr Oscar's identity was severe. He chose the path of least resistance. He gave up, and people around him gave up on him. This is the 'giving in-given up' syndrome. Helplessness and hopelessness are the key features of this phenomenon. Dysthymia is also a possibility. There can be no argument that Mr Oscar was depressed by his losses. The loss of family roles can and does extract a price. For Mr Oscar, the price was isolation, depression, and a profound feeling of disconnection from the people he loved and who loved him, and who ultimately gave purpose and meaning to his life.

CONCLUSION

Loss of family roles is a common experience for people who become chronically ill. The degree of loss is a function of the severity of the condition and the nature and complexity of the particular family dynamics. Responses to loss vary greatly, as observed in the cases discussed in this chapter. Responses to loss may be very complex and include deep sadness, anger, and frustration. Necessary family roles, especially the instrumental ones, are maintained nevertheless by even quite dysfunctional families.

Family losses cover every category of family functioning, from family tasks essential to life to nurturing and support. The families described here were more or less successful in maintaining their necessary family tasks. However, in the affective roles, especially with regard to nurturance and support, we observed significant disruption. The patient's age and the life stage of the family are major contributory factors in explaining how families respond. In the Lynn family, the mother's almost complete withdrawal had a hugely disruptive effect to the detriment of the teenage daughter. The Oscar family suffered no less in face of a family member's loss of health and ability to fulfil role functions. There was a striking difference, however, between the two families. Mrs Lynn's husband played a marginal role in family affairs, whereas in the Oscar family, Mr Oscar and his wife, were almost equally involved in every aspect of family life. Mrs Oscar was able to take over many of Mr Oscar's roles. This was not easy for her by any means, but from the children's point of view there was some continuity. It is also significant that the children in the Oscar family were older and therefore more able to absorb the disruptive effect of parental illness without damage to themselves. In contrast, the teenage daughter in the Lynn family became very distressed and then involved in antisocial activities. Mr Lynn, at first, for professional reasons but also because his anger and resentment of his wife, only nominally filled the gaps created by his sick wife. The necessary instrumental tasks were met, but nurturance and support and life-skills development issues were left unattended. Unlike, Mrs Oscar, who also had a chronically ill spouse, Mr Lynn seemed to lack the will and wherewithal even to begin to consider what his wife's illness required in terms of reassignment of family roles. Both families suffered, but on balance, the Oscar family was far more effective than the Lynn family in readjusting family roles and thereby maintaining the health of the family.

Loss of roles was also somewhat differently perceived by the two who were the sick spouses, Mrs Lynn and Mr Oscar. Mrs Lynn, at the height of her clinical depression, was almost oblivious to the impact her illness was having on the family. As her depression improved, she began to reassume some of her usual family roles. She carried a lot of guilt over what happened to her daughter. At the same time, she also felt that her husband was completely ineffectual. From the very beginning of the period after Mr Oscar became incapacitated he was concerned about his loss of family roles. As already explained, his inability to function to the levels of his own satisfaction led him to more and more withdraw from family roles, and increased his level of sadness.

Both of these families suffered as a result of the illness of one parent. The Oscar family, at least in the short run, remained more intact than the Lynn family. The differences in the responses to the loss of family roles by these patients were significant. To some extent these differences can be on the basis of the quality of the marriage, and the willingness and ability of the well partners to fill the gaps left by the partner who was not well, the life-stage of the family at the time one of its adults became ill, the gender of the patient, and the nature of the illness and disability.

We shall now try to compare the other two cases where the patients and their spouses were older. In both cases, the patients were forced into early retirement because of poor health. Mr Morton's response to his illness is hard to categorize. It was obvious that he still led an active life and that his chronic condition had not affected him in any measurable way. Then what might explain his view of himself overwhelmingly as a suffering and disabled individual? When challenged with the observation that he seemed to be leading a full life, he would smile and then return to talk about the pain and suffering caused by his medical condition. It was almost as if he was claiming that he had a right to be ill. To prove his point he would periodically take himself to his local hospital emergency department, only to be told that there was nothing they could do for him there. Perhaps Mr Morton was unable to accept that there was no cure for his pain. Therefore, he engaged in behaviours that at least confirmed to him that he had an incurable and chronic disease that was interfering with his enjoyment of life. His complaint was a kind of protest. In all other respects, he was living a normal life. It is also noteworthy that his wife played a major role in keeping Mr Morton functional and participating in his family roles.

Mrs Neil, in contrast, was fully accepting of her medical conditions and the associated disability. At the core of her sorrow was her husband's indifference. These two cases are especially important from a clinical perspective. Mrs Neil's response to his wife's health issues were enormously complicated by the family situation. Mr Morton's persistent complaint about his unremitting pain had significant underlying psychological meaning. The reactions of these two individuals to their loss of family roles go beyond the sadness, anger, and other emotions that we commonly associate with loss. Each of these cases revealed major differences in family dynamics that either cushioned or aggravated the psychological responses to the loss of family roles. It must be reiterated that the literature is relatively silent on the topic of loss of family roles. Yet anyone concerned about the psychological health of a chronically ill person will readily recognize the value that family roles are important to people, and be able to imagine how the inability to remain engaged in these roles has far reaching consequences for everyone in the family and certainly for the patient.

Finally, the four cases described in this chapter, when taken together, demonstrate the complex psychological and social factors, apart from the medical ones, that help shape individual responses to chronic illness.

6

Chronic Illness and Sexual Roles

The sexual relationship is generally regarded as an integral part of adult intimacy. Any attempt to separate sexual roles from the more general affection and caring common in any intimate relationship is laden with shortcomings. Yet, many medical conditions such as major depression, diabetes, heart disease, and prostrate conditions, as well as the effects of medications such as anti-hypertensive drugs, or psychological trauma and grief, compromise sexual desire or even eliminate it. Many couples confronted with this problem deal with this loss in a matter of fact way and their relationship does not seem to suffer any adverse consequences. For many others the loss of intimacy and closeness is difficult. Some engage in recrimination, and some use the loss of libido in one partner as an opportunity to disengage from unsatisfactory sexual relations.

Many men equate loss of libido with loss of manhood, and many women with loss of their womanhood. The age of the partners in the couple involved may also influence their response to the loss of their sexual relationship. In short, the response to loss of libido may have no effect or very little effect on a relationship, or it can have enormous consequences. In this chapter, we shall examine some of these effects. Furthermore, through case illustrations we hope to show some of the more complicated responses to the loss of libido as a result of chronic illness and/or disability.

Any painful chronic conditions will likely interfere with the patient's sexual relations. Pain rather than actual loss of libido is what gets in the way of sex for these people. Among those with chronic pain, interference with this aspect of their spousal relationship is pervasive. What is equally true for many of these patients and their partners is that cessation of their sexual relationship is often a prelude to a more global loss of intimacy. Many patients describe their pain as a barrier to intimate relations. However, the absence of sex in a relationship is not universally viewed as a loss. Sometime, it is a resolution to long-existing problems in couples who had been experiencing conflicts in their conjugal relationship. Many men and women patients report that losing the sexual part of their relationship did not amount to any major loss for them. Indeed, chronic illness in general and chronic painful conditions in particular engender so many serious problems that sex is generally given low priority. Nevertheless, as our review will show, loss of sexual function is endemic among persons with chronic pain and other chronic medical conditions. Loss of libido is almost universal in patients with major depressive disorders. Most, if not all, of the studies on depression or other illnesses report a prevalence of sexual problems in their various clinical populations. They do not, however, explore the consequences of loss of sexual relations either on the individual or on these people's relationships. This is a major shortcoming of the literature. We present below a brief literature review on: (1) depression in middle age; (2) medical conditions and depression; (3) chronic pain conditions and depression; (4) physical conditions and sexual dysfunction; and (5) chronic pain and sexual dysfunction. In examining this literature, we offer a fuller appreciation of the combined impact of physical illness and depression on sexual functioning.

DEPRESSION AND MIDDLE AGE

One of the most common symptoms of depression is loss or lowering of libido. Depression, like chronic pain conditions, often has its onset in mid-life. Mid-life is also a time of much personal and family upheaval. For these reason we present this short review.

El-Rufaie and Absood (1993) investigated the prevalence, nature, and severity of depression in 217 Arab subjects, aged sixteen and older. The overall prevalence rate of depression was 27.6 per cent. Morbidity was higher among women than men. The group in the age range of thirty-five to fifty-four years was most susceptible to depression and anxiety-depression, and the overall severity of their disorder was mild to moderate. This paper did not offer any theory to explain the high morbidity in the middle-aged group. Maes et al. (1994) considered a bio-chemical explanation for age variation in depressive illnesses. In a study of 118 patients with major depression and eighty non-depressed control subjects, they found a significant negative correlation between age and cortisol levels in morning plasma samples in control subjects, but not in the depressed group. They concluded that middle age could signal a turning point in the functions of the hypothalamic-pituitary-adrenal axis, differentiating between normal people and those with major depression.

Bromberger and Matthews (1994) investigated the relationship between the employment status of middle-aged women and depression. Their study involved 524 women. They found that non-employed women reported higher levels of depressive symptoms than did employed women. There were larger levels of depression among unemployed women with less education, with low support from family and friends, and with low levels of marital satisfaction; this last factor was the most symptomatic. The authors concluded that with respect to mood, paid work had a beneficial effect on the mental health of middle-aged women.

A study involving 102 middle-aged women investigating the impact of their mother's death was undertaken by Moss et al. (1993). The sudden death of the mother caused more intense grief, accompanied by less acceptance and more thoughts of reunion than when the deaths of the mother occurred in a nursing home. This study measured depression, grief, somatic symptoms, impact on the sense of self, degree of acceptance of the death, and the quality of ties with the mother. The findings were complex, as many of these reactions were intercorrelated. Nevertheless, they were differentially associated with the characteristics of the daughter and the mother, and the quality of their relationship.

In another investigation, involving women aged between the early forties and early fifties, Helson and Wink (1992) reported that normative personality changes in these women were not interrupted by menopausal status, 'empty nest' syndrome, or involvement in caring for parents. Around age forty, however, many women experience turmoil. This study is important in supporting the view that from a psychological perspective, middle age is not necessarily a period of increased vulnerability for emotional distress.

Gallo and colleagues (1993), in a very different kind of study, examined the risk factors for the onset of depression in middle age and later life. Subjects with a history of major depression were excluded. Of their subjects aged forty years and older, there were 180 incident cases, and 960 subjects at risk for future occurrence of major depression. Risk of depression for those who were employed was not significantly different than for those who were not employed. But those who had twelve years of schooling were at less risk for depression than less who did not complete high school.

This brief incursion into the midlife-depression literature suggests that the evidence is equivocal. Depression may occur in middle age, and the reason for this may be biochemical or grief or significant demographic factors. Yet, there is also evidence supporting the hypothesis that this phase in life may not render one specifically vulnerable to depressive disorders.

CHRONIC PAIN AND DEPRESSION

The presence of chronic pain, however, seems to alter this absence of vulnerability depression in middle age to a substantial degree. The body of literature on pain and depression is so large as to deserve a major review. Indeed, several such reviews were conducted during the 1980s, and the general conclusion was that while depression was not uncommon in patients with idiopathic chronic pain, it was not inevitable. There was a major shift away from equating chronic pain without organic cause with depressive disorders. Three facts emerged: (1) A proportion of chronic pain patients also suffer from major depression. (2) Negative life events, events associated with mid-life and financial hardships, in conjunction with unremitting pain cause many patients to become sad and discouraged. (3) Many patients with chronic pain were not depressed, although many of their symptoms such as low energy, low libido, and sleep disturbance overlapped with symptoms of depression.

It would be erroneous, however, to suppose that the debate is over. A quick glance at a more recent literature review perpetuates the contradictions and confusion. Ruoff (1996) claimed that 50 per cent of chronic pain sufferers also suffer from depression as co-morbidity. His claim further suggested that both depression and chronic pain share common biological pathways. Aggressive treatment with the new generation of antidepressants is strongly recommended. Eisendrath (1995) noted that many chronic pain conditions are associated with known psychiatric disorders such as somatization disorder, hypochondriasis, factitious physical illnesses, and pain associated with psychosocial problems. Here, we have two alternate, yet overlapping views of depression and psychiatric problems and chronic pain. One claims common biological pathways for pain and depression, the other claims chronic pain to be a primary psychiatric disorder. They are, of course, not mutually exclusive.

McGuigan (1995) found that psychosocial factors were involved in the depression of chronic pain sufferers. Banks and Kerns (1996), in their extensive review of the pain and depression literature, concluded that the unique experience of living with chronic pain may account for the high prevalence of depression.

Overestimation of depression in the chronic pain population was observed in a Finnish study (Estlander, Takala, and Verkasalo, 1995). The researchers of this report concluded that a diagnosis of depression based on a sum score of an inventory that contains somatic-vegetative signs of depression (inventories on depressions almost always include somatic-vegetative signs) may lead to this overestimation of depression. Even this short incursion into the current literature suggests unresolved diagnostic issues. This debate is likely to continue until such time that more objective laboratory-based investigation for major depression become available. The fact, however, remains that chronic illness accompanied by depression further complicates sexual relationships.

CHRONIC ILLNESS AND DEPRESSION

The literature on chronic illness and depression is truly voluminous. We present three recent comprehensive reports to show the high rate of prevalence of depression and other psychological problems in the chronically ill population. An Icelandic study based on a representative survey of 825 adult residents (twenty to seventy years of age), of the urban Reyjavik area, found that chronic physical conditions involved depression directly, as well as indirectly by aggravating domestic, occupational, and economic strains, and by undermining personal resources (Vilhjalmsson et al., 1998). Chronic illness posed a real threat to self-esteem and compromised any sense of mastery.

Rethelyi, Berghammer, and Kopp (2001), in a Hungarian study, investigated the prevalence of pain symptoms causing disabilities in day-to-day living and their connection to depressive symptoms. A representative sample of 12,640 adults participated in a door-to-door survey. Pain prevalence was estimated at 32.7 per cent. Among those reporting pain, 30.2 per cent reported depressive symptoms. There were demographic variables influencing the rate of prevalence for pain together with depression. However, for the purpose of this chapter, this study lends further credence that pain and depression coexist in a significant segment of pain sufferers, and it is reasonable to assume that in this population diminution in libido may not be uncommon.

In a comprehensive literature review on emotional disorder in patients with chronic physical illness, Guthrie (1996) found that the psychological reaction to any physical disorder was transitional, moving from initial shock to gradual adjustment. However, adjustment disorders, anxiety states, and depressive states were common consequences of physical illness. Studies included in this review were randomized controlled trials of at least six week's duration and had thirty or more subjects. On this basis, fourteen studies met the criteria for inclusion in this review. The point of note is that chronic illness, while by itself capable of compromising sexual potency, is even further compromised by the presence of depression.

PHYSICAL ILLNESS AND SEXUAL DYSFUNCTION

In a major investigation of psychological, physical, and social problems in relation to sexual dysfunction, 789 men and 979 women responded to a mailed questionnaire (Dunn, Croft and Hackett 1999). In general terms, sexual dysfunction in men was attributed to self-reported physical problems and women to self-reported psychological and social problems. Erectile problems were commonly associated with prostrate problems, hypertension, and diabetes. All female sexual problems were associated with anxiety and depression.

There appears to be an underestimation of sexual problems in women, even those with diabetes (Ertekin, 1998). Newman and Bertelson (1986) interviewed eighty-one women with insulin-treated diabetes and found that thirty-eight subjects presented with sexual dysfunction and forty-three did not. The more frequently reported sexual difficulties were inhibited sexual excitement, inhibited sexual desire, and dyspareunia. These subjects were more depressed, more stereotypical in their sex roles, and less satisfied with their sexual relationships than those without sexual problems. This study lent further credence to the idea that psychological, social, and physical problems combined accentuated sexual dysfunction.

In a six-year follow-up study of fifty women and fifty-one men who were insulin-treated diabetics, significantly higher prevalence of sexual dysfunction was found among the men with signs of peripheral neuropathy (Jensen, 1986). Some subjects recovered from their sexual problems during the intervening period without any therapeutic interventions. Once again, a combination of psychological factors combined with the level of acceptance of disease revealed a strong correlation with sexual dysfunction.

Sexual problems associated with heart diseases and arthritic disorders have also come under scrutiny. An investigation of sixteen women and two men attending an out-patient psychiatric clinic compared them with twelve patients with arthritis and twelve patients with heart conditions (Bouras, Vanger and Bridges, 1986). The findings were consistent relative to the very different marital profiles for the three groups. As for sexual problems, the depressed group was the most affected, cardiac patients were least dissatisfied, and the arthritic patients fell somewhere in-between.

One problem often reported by arthritic patients is the underinvestigation of their sexual difficulties. One hundred and eighty six out-patients with arthritic disorders were asked if they would like their sexual problems to be part of routine medical examination (Blake et al., 1986). Only 22 per cent reported that a physician had ever inquired into their sexual problems, but a remarkable 77 per cent felt that such an inquiry would be helpful. This study provides indirect evidence for preponderance of sexual problems among patients with chronic illness.

CHRONIC PAIN AND SEXUAL DYSFUNCTION

We have presented a very brief review to show that medical problems and sexual difficulties often go hand in hand. To reiterate what was stated earlier, this body of literature provides very little insight into the question of perceptions of loss associated with sexual dysfunction. In the context of chronic pain conditions, which generally tend to afflict middle-aged persons, sexual problems tend to be endemic.

Roy (1989) in an in-depth investigation of family functioning with respect to thirty-two chronic back pain and headache sufferers found pervasive loss of sexual functioning in this population. Some of the early studies involving patients with physical disabilities (Peterson, 1979) and organic conditions (Katz, 1969; Montenero and Donatone, 1962; Rubin and Babbott, 1958; Schoffling, 1963) found high levels of sexual and relationship problems.

Some of the earlier studies clearly established sexual difficulties to be a common problem among chronic pain patients (Flor, Turk, and Scholz, 1987; Hudgens, 1979; Maruta and Osborne, 1978). More recent literature is reviewed briefly to assess the current state of knowledge. One point of note is that contemporary studies are more complex than the earlier ones. For instance, Monga et al. (1999), in an investigation of forty-five chronic back pain patients, found that not only was sexual function compromised in a majority of them, but many reported finding some satisfaction from fantasizing about sex, although they had a fear of aggravating their pain by actually engaging in sexual acts. Special positions, such as sitting on a chair during intercourse, enabled some patients to continue to maintain some measure of sexual activity.

The significance of psychological factors was noted in a study of seventy chronic pain patients (Monga et al., 1998). This study failed to establish any relationship between severity of pain, duration of intercourse, frequency of intercourse, and sexual functioning. A significant relationship was found between disability status, age, and significantly, several psychological variables.

In a comparative study of sexual functioning of cancer patients with chronic pain sufferers, Tan and colleagues (1998) found that the age of a patient was a determining factor in frequency, drive, and satisfaction with sexual activities. The greater the age in these two populations, the lower their level of sexual activity. Significantly, pain itself did not differentiate the two groups in their satisfaction with sex.

The final study in this section involved sixty-five women with interstitial cystitis (a painful disease with urinary urgency) whose sexual function was investigated (Rose, 1997). Results showed that pre-morbid level of sexual satisfaction, sexual communication, range of sexual experiences, positive affect, and sexual drive predicted sexual satisfaction. However, pain alone emerged as a significant negative predictor. Many women preserved their sexuality through the practice of non-intercourse activities, but also through love, intimacy, and affection. The scope of this study surpassed the traditional focus on the narrow aspect of sexual intercourse to the broader issues of intimacy and affection. For that reason alone, the findings of this study are of particular interest to us.

Summary

The literature review suggests that chronic illness directly compromises sexual functioning, and is further complicated by the presence of depression. This depression can be a reaction to the vicissitudes of chronic illness, or it may have an independent presence (co-morbidity). We also examined briefly the depression and mid-life literature, as many chronic pain conditions occur in mid-life, is also the case with depressive disorders. The presence of depression vastly complicates the sexual functioning and must be taken into account in the assessment of loss of sexual desire.

Depression and many chronic physical conditions go hand in hand. Depression also has a very profound impact on libido and loss of sexual desire is common. When this is considered in combination with chronic pain and other medical conditions, which for complex medical reasons, lower or even eliminate sexual drive, we can begin to appreciate the magnitude of the problem. Our brief exploration of the literature on depression as well as physical conditions shows that sexual functioning easily is at risk in the presence of medical conditions, and when combined with depression, that risk is substantially enhanced.

In the case studies that follow we hope to show that the loss of sexual desire has many faces and has many levels of complexity. We have deliberately chosen cases which show that the loss of sexual role may only partly be accounted for by the medical condition, while it is frequently complicated by psychological, psychiatric and social factors.

TOO MUCH TO BEAR: MS. PETERS

Ms. Peters (see Chapter 9) was in her teens when she sought help at our clinic and thus, by virtue of her young age, represents an exception to our general rule for case reports in this book. She was referred to the pain clinic because of her chronic lower abdominal pain following hysterectomy and vaginoplasty. Apart from the pain, these surgeries had a profound effect on the patient and her parents, and to a lesser degree on her older brother. Collectively, all members of the family perceived an enormous sense of loss, which over time, they were able to articulate as centring on Ms. Peters's ensuing infertility.

This family had emigrated to Canada from South America when the children were very young. The parents were deeply religious. Ms. Peters shared her parents values and had come to believe that her serious illness and the subsequent surgeries, which had left her permanently scarred, were divine retribution for something or other. She was altogether unsure of the reasons for her perceived punishment, for she had always been a good person and followed her parents' guidance.

Ms. Peters felt no sense of belonging – this is especially serious in teenagers – with her peers at school. She felt different from the others. While she was in hospital, several of the children she had come to know there died. There were other children in the hospital who were very ill. She felt that she had grown up too soon too fast. She felt that her peers at school seemed to be preoccupied with superficial things. She did not have one person to whom she could relate and share her thoughts and feelings. Her best friend was her mother.

What did Ms. Peters think about her surgeries? For one thing, she would now not be able to have children. She could not understand why she should be deprived so. The operation had left her feeling less than a woman as she was beginning to become a woman. This was just not fair. Her parents never said anything, but she knew that they were disappointed that she would never have a baby. Did she cry about this loss? Only when she was alone. She also felt that she was not very attractive, and now this. Perhaps, that was the reason why no one bothered with her at school.

Ms. Peters actually drew a picture of her predicament. The picture was entirely black showing a black blob in the middle surrounded by thick black walls. She explained that the black blob in the middle was herself, and she had no way out. This was a telling portrayal of her state of mind, and how she felt entirely alone and without hope. Did this picture have to do with the loss of her uterus? That was only part of the answer. She felt all alone. She just did not belong, and she thought she was the cause of much of the rift between her parents. She often heard them arguing. They had hardly ever argued before she got sick.

Analysis

A threat, a challenge, a blow, all these terms can be interchangeably used to describe Ms. Peters's feelings about her identity. She had been irrevocably changed. This, happening at a critical phase of her development, when her sense of womanhood was just beginning to take root. Her conflict around her peer relations, which manifested as both wanting and not wanting to be a part of her peer group, feeling unattractive, and divine retribution can be understood in the context of her developmental stage. They confirm her sense of being different as well as bad. In her mind, Ms. Peters tried to fight the loss of her reproductive organs by trying to minimize it. She could adopt not one but many children when she grew up, and she would like to be a pediatrician and help sick children.

However, just beneath the surface was the overwhelming feeling of having been cheated of her womanhood, letting down her family, and surely being different than her peers – who she thought were all better looking than her, and yet still had their uteri intact. We have previously discussed the effects of hysterectomy on women in general, and there is consensus that many women regard this surgery as a threat to their core identity as a woman. These responses vary based on age, personality, personal circumstances, and so on.

For a young teenager, this particular loss is likely to have considerable poignancy. Unfortunately, the literature is silent on this topic and there is always the risk of drawing too many generalized conclusions based on a single case.

What, however, is undeniable is that Ms. Peters's emerging sexual identity was under severe strain. Curiously, she never asked the question of 'Why me?' Rather, she viewed this as divine retribution for reasons that were far from self-evident. This perspective only added to her heightened sense of guilt and 'badness' which made even her parents fall out. She was engulfed in her 'badness.' Self-recrimination was the driving force. Ms. Peters was in a state of mourning. She was taken into therapy, and at the time of this writing, is making progress.

Ms. Peters's family situation and the collective response by the parents and her brother to her surgeries was great sadness. This had very serious consequences for our young patient, and contributed to her feelings of guilt. Her mother tried to maintain a very positive attitude, and was indeed our patient's main source of support. From time to time, though, even the mother succumbed to despair, depression, and guilt over daughter's loss of reproductive organs. The entire family system was in the throes of grief, and this had gone on for quite some time. Our approach to deal with this loss was to persuade the family to consider the reasons behind the surgeries and what the consequences might have been without them. Somehow, this simple reality had become buried under their overwhelming sense of loss and grief, complicated at it was by guilt.

Ms. Peters's critical developmental stage, the family's reaction to her surgeries, their collective belief in divine retribution, and the very nature of the loss, namely, her ability to ever have babies, contributed to making this situation very grievous indeed.

'SEX IS NOT FOR ME' – MS. QUILL

Ms. Quill, a rather shy woman, made this stark statement to her therapist during their very first session together. She had been referred for unremitting pelvic pain following the onset and treatment of endometriosis. Her pain was regarded as secondary to her disease. Ms. Quill's childhood history was one of chaos. She was the youngest of five sisters. Her father was a farmer and her mother a homemaker. The father was an alcoholic and regularly beat his wife in front of the children. Seeing her mother being physically and verbally abused was among Ms. Quill's earliest childhood memories. She was unable to recall a single happy event or memory from her childhood.

When Ms. Quill was still very young, her mother unable to tolerate the abuse, left home. Her father immediately sought the custody of the children and silenced them with threats. In fact, he forced the oldest child to sign an affidavit saying that the father neither drank nor was abusive. Thus, the father was awarded custody of the children. This event had profound effects on the children's attitude towards the father. To this day, he maintains some kind of control over our patient. She continues to feel uncomfortable in his presence. She would like to confront him about the past, but feels that she lacks the courage to do so, and in any event, he would deny that any abuse took place. In the meantime, three of the five children have a very close relationship with the mother.

At about age fourteen Ms. Quill became involved with drugs and alcohol. At age fifteen, with grade 8 behind her, she ran away from home and soon after married a man who was then nineteen years old and had a baby. Before too long her husband started physically and sexually abusing her, and she divorced him after about four years of marriage. Following the divorce, she had sexual relations with numerous men and continued to abuse drugs and alcohol. Then she moved to another city, and lived rough for a while until she was able to obtain work at a bar as an exotic dancer. She made good money and slowly gained some semblance of control over her life. During this time she also met a married man and fell in love; this liaison lasted four years. On reflection, Ms. Quill felt that this was the only significant relationship she had ever had, as this man's kindness to her was something she had never experienced before.

Despite the relative stability in her life during this period, which lasted about five years, she had a lot of guilt about her occupation as an exotic dancer. She stated that she never truly got used to removing her clothes in front of 'leering' men. Nevertheless, she was able to stay away from drugs and prostitution which she knew to be common among her friends and fellow workers. Her friendship with the married man had run its course, and she was beginning to feel unwell. As well, she was becoming increasingly despondent about her work. She decided to return to her hometown. Soon after, she was diagnosed with endometriosis.

She made drastic changes in her lifestyle. She became a teetotaller and decided to get her high school diploma. In the meantime, she found employment as a home care worker. Ms. Quill continued to harbour considerable shame and guilt over her past life, and began to isolate herself socially. She had not had any sexual liaison with men since she parted company with her married friend. Other than work and visits with her mother, she became housebound, and complained of great unease in any kind of social situations.

Analysis

Ms. Quill's dramatic change in her attitude to sex and in her lifestyle preceded the onset of endometriosis. This, of course, is a very painful disorder, and the pain is often exacerbated during intercourse. Pelvic and lower abdominal pain is not un-common in patients with this disease. Ms. Quill's decision to terminate all relationships with men has to be understood against this background. Her one meaningful relationship, where she had felt loved and valued, was with a married man. Upon termination of this relationship, she returned to her hometown and changed her life.

It would be hard to underestimate the impact of Ms. Quill's disease on her attitude towards men in general and sex in par-ticular. Unlike the previous patient, Ms. Quill presented a very matter-of-fact explanation for her disease. She was just unlucky and many women get it. The absence of guilt or any attribution to 'badness' for her disease was noticeable. Yet, she did have a lot of guilt and, indeed, shame regarding the kind of life she had led until recently. Her withdrawal from the social world could not be explained any other way. She did not use her disease to interfere with matters of import to her. She managed to upgrade her education and find socially responsible work.

What is noteworthy is that Ms. Quill's lack of interest in sex was tantamount to lack of interest in men. In a case like this, it would be relatively easy to attribute her lack of interest in sex to her disease. That is the point of the story. It would be impos-sible to understand Ms. Quill's transformation without an ad-equate appreciation of her personal history. Loss of sexual in-terest and possible infertility was not seen by her as a personal loss. Rather, she had embarked on a course of 'cleansing' her body and mind, and her disease undoubtedly accelerated and solidified this transformation.

SEX AND LOVE: MR ROPER

Mr Roper was referred to our pain clinic following an employ-ment-related injury to his back. He worked in the building trade, doing heavy labour. Before his most recent accident he had had serious problems with his knees for which he had had several surgeries.

Mr Roper had emigrated at a young age to Canada. He faced serious discrimination because of his national origin. As a young man he constantly got into brawls, drank too much, and generally lived a rather unruly life. Through all of this he worked in the building trade. He managed, to a degree, to overcome some of his turbulent behaviour, got married, and had three children. His first marriage ended in divorce, and he was most reluctant to discuss the reasons for this divorce. His attitude was one of defiance. Anyone who did not like his ways was free to leave. He felt under no obligation to anyone.

He was now in a new relationship, which had become quite problematic. Mr Roper was given to extreme outbursts of temper which his partner understandably found very intimidating. However, he had never laid a finger on her, or even verbally abused her. He gave very little outward evidence of caring or loving his partner. His partner described herself as very demonstrative and giving. She was afraid to complain about his apparent lack of love for her, because on one or two occasions when she had done so, she had been told that she was under no obligation to stay in the relationship. Any sexual relationship between this couple had ceased within the first year of their relationship. Mr Roper expressed no sense of loss about the absence of sex. His partner, on the other hand, not only missed sex, but also any kind of intimacy.

Analysis

It would be virtually impossible to explain Mr Roper's attitude to love and sex without some understanding of his past. He was very reluctant to reveal very much about his past, other than to leave an impression that he had learned not to trust anyone and to avoid emotional involvement, lest he should be hurt. Over the years he had built an emotional moat around himself, and no one in his orbit was allowed to cross it. Much of his behaviour had to be understood in the context of a harsh childhood and very troubled adolescence. His singular failure to enter into and maintain adult reciprocal relationships had very little or nothing to do with his medical conditions. He never invoked his physical pain as a reason for avoiding any intimacy with his partner. Rather, his attitude was one of defiance which seemed to communicate 'take me as you find me, but don't try to change me.'

Underneath Mr Roper's manifest anger and hostility was a sad and depressed person who seemed to inhabit a sad and hostile world. This is a particularly poignant case because it illustrates how loss of intimacy and loss of sexual functioning are not necessarily casualties of disease and pain, although frequently they are, but rather how a complex and mainly painful past may have a profound effect in shaping a man's personality. Mr Roper's inability to trust anyone, combined with his fear of intimacy, could in large measure, explain not only abstinence from sex but also his inability to express or accept affection in his relationship.

A CASE OF SEXUAL ABUSE? – MRS SEMPLE

Mrs Semple had a very complicated medical history. She was born with a congenital hip problem and had bilateral prosthetic replacement. Unfortunately, the correction did not take place until the fourth year of her life, which left her with difficulty in walking and in chronic pain. She had corrective surgeries, but later she fractured one hip, which had to be replaced. She used a shoulder crutch for walking. She had unrelenting pain in the lower back region and suffered from severe bouts of muscle contraction headaches.

Mrs Semple's family history was complicated. Her childhood memories were mixed. As a sick child she received special attention from both her parents, and she was convinced that this had coloured her relationship with her siblings forever. Her parents did not get along. Her father was an alcoholic and engaged in occasionally physical, but most verbal abuse of his wife and the other children. He was, however, very protective of his sick child, and thus our patient enjoyed a very special relationship with him. Nevertheless, she became very resentful of his drinking and abusive behaviour as she gained insight into his conduct towards her mother and siblings.

Mrs Semple had virtually no experience with dating and married the first man who showed any interest in her. It did not take her very long to discover that her husband was very controlling, non-communicative, and emotionally unresponsive. She did not regard his behaviour as abusive, but rather as unpleasant. He was also an excellent provider.

Very early in the marriage Mrs Semple became anorexic, her weight dropping down to 74 pounds. Her husband was seemingly unconcerned about her declining health. They had two children, a boy and a girl, in quick succession. Children brought some stability to her life. But her problems assumed serious proportions as the children grew older and became less dependent on her. Her sense of being controlled by her husband became overwhelming. She could do nothing without his permission. He would demand a detailed account of her activities when he returned home from his business trips. After some time, she concluded that she was not only controlled by this man, but that he was emotionally abusing her.

As stated at the outset, Mrs Semple had serious health issues and lived with much pain. She had restricted movements of her hips and legs. Regardless of her health status, her husband demanded regular sexual contact. He was unwilling to consider anything other than sex in the conventional position of the man being on top. Mrs Semple found these sexual experiences not only unbearably painful, but entirely humiliating for his total lack of consideration combined with his denial of her health problems.

At the same time, she was driven by her sense of duty and obligation to give in to his, what amounted to, cruel demands. This was the situation that persisted for many years. Mrs Quill debated the pros and cons of leaving this man, but her insecurity about her own health and the fear of living alone usually won out. Their children grew up and left home. After twenty years of living in an untenable situation, Mrs Quill finally left her husband.

Analysis

Mrs Semple's story is one of great loss and regret. She had enormous sadness about her marriage. It had been loveless. She not only never experienced enjoyable sex, even when her health was relatively good, but she had been deprived of any sense of intimacy and love in her only relationship with a partner. It must be understood that Mrs Semple's multiple physical problems made sexual intercourse very painful for her. Her flexibility was very restricted, and her anorexia had left her in a very weakened state and without much sexual desire. She viewed herself as sexually undesirable. Yet she longed for intimacy.

Her total financial dependence on her husband had made her feel obliged to give in to his demands for sex. He often demanded sex as his right and her duty. Mrs Semple had a vague notion that her husband was being unreasonable, while having the right to sex, but could only explain his behaviour in terms of his total disregard for his wife's wishes and feelings. Mr Quill was, at best, unkind. It is very difficult to see his total lack of sympathy and even simple human consideration for his wife's medical state as reasonable in any way. Mrs Semple was in an emotionally and sexually abusive situation. The sexual and intimate parts of her marriage remained unfulfilled for her.

CONCLUSION

Loss of sexual desire is not uncommon in relation to chronic illness. This could be a direct consequence of the disease itself, such as in the case of diabetes and major trauma, or it could be related to depression, which is common in the chronically ill population. Many patients have a very clear sense of loss about their diminished or absent sexual needs or their inability to engage in pleasurable sex because of their physical limitations and pain. Many patients and their partners find new and novel ways to maintain their connection and intimacy through experimentation with sex, discovering new and comfortable positions for coitus, or other ways of giving each other sexual pleasure. For many patients and their partners sex falls by the wayside and tends to have low priority.

We deliberately chose cases to show the complexity of the issues associated with loss of sexual functions. Our first case, that of a teenager, gave us an understanding of the grief for the whole family as this young woman lost her reproductive organs as a result of necessary surgery. Grief combined with guilt created a family environment characterized by parental conflict and individual isolation. Our second case, a young woman with endometriosis is a story of penitence and regrets enormously complicated by childhood events. The third case concerns a man who is unable to share affection, part of which is a sexual relationship with his partner, for complex reasons of rejection and anger. Our final case is clearly one of unfulfilled longings and emotional and even sexual abuse of a woman with seriously compromised health. Collectively these patient stories depict the intricate nature of the loss of sexual desire or fulfilment and the equally intricate reactions to this loss.

7

Old Age, Pain, and Loss

Chronic pain is often accompanied by a variety of losses. These may include job loss, loss of mobility, losses associated with parental and spousal roles, loss of social roles, and many others (Roy, 2001). Losses also occur at a personal or existential level, affecting the individual's self and personal control (Kelly, 1998). These losses add significantly to a patient's sense of hopelessness and may even lead to depression. Depression and depressive symptoms are relatively common in persons with chronic pain.

There exists a notion that a common accompaniment of old age is pain. Chronic diseases abound in old age as do certain kinds of aches and intermittent pain. For instance, joint pain is common in the elderly, while headaches are less frequent. In fact, elderly persons take pain so much for granted that they are far too accepting even of relatively severe pain, and frequently fail to seek treatment.

Old age is characterized by a multitude and variety of losses. Loss of health, loss through the death of one's spouse and friends, loss of mobility, and loss of financial security, and so on are all losses experienced by many adults as they leave middle age. However, it is also a statistical fact that more variability in health status is to be found in the elderly population than in any other age group. Healthy women and men who are eighty-five years old are no longer hard to find. Yet, to a large degree, most people are dead long before they attain that great age. Among those people who are eighty-five years old, we will also find an assortment of chronic disorders.

Against this background we shall present two cases. The first is of an elderly woman, Mrs Thomas. She has chronic pain and other ailments, including breast cancer. She has experienced severe additional losses, including the sudden death of her son at age forty-five and the death of her husband soon after his institutionalization because of Alzheimer's disease. To help us arrive at an understanding of Mrs Thomas, her capacity for survival, and the relevance of loss, caregiving, and family issues to her pain management and pain management in older adults generally, we include a review of some of the relevant literature.

A SURVIVOR? – MRS THOMAS

We begin this discussion with a brief history of our patient who was in her seventies when she first presented at our clinic. Her husband's diagnosis of Alzheimer's disease and his subsequent hospitalization, her own breast cancer, and the sudden death of her only child, a middle-aged son, occurred while she was our patient.

Mrs Thomas was referred to the pain clinic with back complaints. She had had a fall, injuring her eighth rib. The computer-assisted tomographic (CAT) scan showed a compression fracture at L4, possible spinal stenosis at this level, and a disc bulging at L4. Mrs Thomas was experiencing difficulty with walking and reported being in constant pain. She also suffered from lupus.

Mrs Thomas's psychosocial history on arrival at our clinic was not without complexity. She was confronted with two problems. Her husband had recently been diagnosed with Alzheimer's disease and was showing early signs of confusion and memory loss. Second, her own declining health had become an obstacle in her ability to function at a reasonable level. An added complication arose in relation to her son and only child. He was married with two young children, and his relationship with this patient had its difficulties. The son was very close to his father, and at times expressed concern over the father's well-being, to Mrs Thomas's chagrin. She received very little practical help from either her son or the daughter-in-law. The son did not make a very good living and from time to time Mrs Thomas had felt obliged to bail him out financially.

Over the next two years the condition of Mrs Thomas's husband deteriorated to a point where he was becoming physically violent towards her. At about this time she herself was diagnosed with breast cancer. Her attitude towards this new development was close to indifference. She was almost totally preoccupied with her husband and with what might be the best course of action for his care. Mrs Thomas showed an extraordinary level of ambivalence about institutionalizing her husband. Her son was strongly opposed to this idea, although he provided very little day-to-day help towards his care. Eventually Mr Thomas was placed in a nursing home. Very suddenly and unexpectedly the son died from a brain hemorrhage a year later. We shall focus on the following key issues in Mrs Thomas's life: (1) pain in old age, (2) her husband's Alzheimer's disease, (3) the death of her son, (4) family issues, and (5) loss and grieving issues.

CHRONIC PAIN IN OLD AGE

Pain in old age was until recently a pretty much neglected topic. This has changed, and at present this topic is receiving considerable attention from researchers. One entire issue of *Pain Research and Management* (2001) was devoted to pain and aging. It is estimated that approximately 30 per cent of individuals between the ages twenty-five and thirty-four, 50 per cent of those between forty-five and fifty-four, and over 60 per cent of those aged seventy-five years or older are afflicted with chronic pain problems (Elliott et al., 1999). Mrs Thomas had lived with considerable pain even before her fall which culminated in her referral to the pain clinic. But older adults are not frequently referred to pain clinics (Harkins, Kwentus, and Price, 1984).

Oriol (1991) observed that under-representation of older people in pain clinics has been attributed to age-related stoicism, negative referral biases, and the stigma facing chronic pain sufferers. Gagliese and Melzack (1997) examined three factors that may contribute to inadequate treatment of geriatric pain patients: (1) inadequate pain assessment; (2) mismanagement of pain because of the possible adverse effects of pharmacological treatment and the almost total absence of psychological intervention, and; (3) misconceptions about pain and aging such as higher thresholds for pain tolerance in the elderly, as well as the idea that pain is a given in old age.

There is some empirical evidence to support the notion that older persons tend to be accepting of pain symptoms. In a study of healthy and well-functioning elderly individuals living in the community, one key finding was the willingness of these people to live with a surprisingly high level of pain (Roy and Thomas, 1988). Their attitude to pain was in part explained by the fact that this group of elderly subjects viewed themselves as healthy, and indeed most of them were engaged in a variety of physical and social activities. Stoller and Forster (1994) found that pain symptoms in the elderly did not inevitably result in them seeking a medical consultation. Rather, it was their uncertainty about the seriousness of the pain and its possible causes, in combination with how it interfered with their activities that prompted them to seek medical help. Cook and Thomas (1994) confirmed the limited role of pain symptoms as a predictor of health care utilization by older adults. Cook and Roy (1995), in a review study of the beliefs and attitudes of the elderly towards pain symptoms, concluded that some elderly people show considerable courage and endurance in tolerating severe aches and pains and sometimes demonstrate an almost a fatalistic attitude towards living with pain.

PREVALENCE OF PAIN IN THE ELDERLY

How common is pain among elderly people? A significant body of literature has emerged addressing this question, and in the process is demystifying many misperceptions about the prevalence of pain complaints in the elderly. Joint pain is more common in the elderly compared with other age groups (Roy and Thomas, 1988; Sternbach 1986). The overall prevalence of pain symptoms in the elderly ranges from 22 per cent to 58 per cent. Although musculoskeletal pain is more common in the elderly, research has consistently shown declining pain complaints with rising age (Anderson et al., 1996; Gibson and Helme, 1995; Moss, Lawton, and Glicksman, 1991).

Rheumatic pain is commonly found in the elderly. Demlow, Liang, and Eaton (1986) reported that such pain was present in 80 per cent of an elderly population studied by them. Roy, Thomas, and Berger (1990), in a comparative study of healthy community-based elderly people and a pain clinic sample of elderly people, found that back and joint pain accounted for 75 per cent and just over 95 per cent of the pain complaints, respectively, in these two populations. One important finding was that the pain in the community sample was much less intense than in the pain clinic sample. Valkenberg (1988) found with a younger population that 30 per cent of men and 55 per cent of women over the age of fifty-five in his sample reported some form of peripheral joint pain. In nursing home samples, the reported range of pain prevalence is between 70 per cent and 83 per cent (Roy and Thomas, 1986; Ferrell, Ferrell, and Osterweil, 1990; Parmelee, Katz, and Lawton, 1991; Sengstaken and King, 1993).

Although pain and old age has a complex relationship, and old age in itself is not sufficient cause for increased pain, certain painful medical conditions are indeed more prevalent in old age, and many diseases also tend to be of late onset (Ferrell, Gibson, and Helme, 1996; Thomas and Roy, 1999; Melanson and Downe-Walmboldt, 1995). Vascular diseases, neurological degenerative conditions, cancer, herpes-zoster, and collagen and bone diseases are more associated with old age (Rowe and Besdine, 1982; Kwentus, Harkins, Lignon, and Silverman, 1985; Melding, 1991). This brief overview shows the prevalence and common pain conditions in the elderly population. It also dispels the notion that pain is a natural accompaniment of old age or that prevalence of pain increases with age. In relation to Mrs Thomas, the chronic pain that commenced with a fall which culminated in chronic joint pain and pain in her rib, complicated by her history of lupus and breast cancer of recent onset. Her overall clinical picture was indeed complex, although not uncommon in the elderly who often report multiple health problems.

FAMILY ISSUES

Mrs Thomas's family problems were certainly not unique. She and her husband had enjoyed a reasonably trouble-free relationship, although in the early days of their marriage, Mr Thomas had been given to angry outbursts. His temper had improved over the years. They had very different interests. She enjoyed art and literature, while his major interest was sports. The situation altered completely with the admission of Mr Thomas to a nursing home. Mrs Thomas was now living alone, which she did not seem to mind. Yet, she complained incessantly about her son's lack of concern for her. She had no regard for her daughter-in-law, and the feelings were mutual. Mrs Thomas was very fond of her three grandchildren and saw them on a regular basis. That changed once her son died, and the daughter-in-law severed virtually all connections with Mrs Thomas, which included access to the grandchildren.

In essence, Mrs Thomas became a widow in rather poor health and with no family support. This is not an unusual situation for the elderly. At the time of her arrival at the pain clinic, Mrs Thomas and her husband were seen together for the purpose of a family assessment, but the venture was dropped after one session, as Mr Thomas was unable to participate in any meaningful way. The only other family contact of the clinic was with the son, who had serious doubts about the level of disability of his mother. From the very beginning, the family problem centred on the question of Mr Thomas's long-term care, and the therapy was focused on Mrs Thomas's ambivalence about the prospect of his institutionalization. In this sense Mrs Thomas's family issues were very different from the more commonly encountered problems of relationships brought on by the emergence of chronic pain problem in one partner of a couple.

Studies of families of the elderly from a systemic point of view are few. The literature on elderly families, however, covers a broad range of problematic areas. Field and colleagues (1993), in a longitudinal study involving sixty-two subjects between seventy-four and ninety-three years of age, found that subjects in better health had more contacts with family members than did those in poorer health. An Indian study involving 720 retired men found that life satisfaction was derived from activities associated with their occupation, hobbies, friends, and voluntary organizations (Mishra, 1992). Religious and household activities and interaction with family members and neighbours had no such impact on life satisfaction. McCamish-Svensson et al. (1999), in a recent Swedish longitudinal study, examined the relationship between family and friends, social supports, health, and life satisfaction for a single cohort of 212 people who were in their eighties. They found that neither the support of children nor friends was related to life satisfaction at either age eighty or eighty-three. Health satisfaction and satisfaction with sibling contact were related to overall life satisfaction at age eighty-three only. They concluded that social support and life satisfaction were complex and multidimensional.

Nevertheless, there is evidence that support from family members is often crucial for the well-being of the elderly. A large-scale Dutch survey of 3,390, subjects between fifty-five and eighty-nine years of age found that older adults not currently involved in a partner relationship were lonelier than older adults who had a partner (Peters and Liefbroer, 1997). Loneliness also increased with the dissolution of relationships. Loss or lack of a partner was more detrimental for males. This suggests that it is difficult to compensate for the lack or loss of a partner relationship, especially for males. An earlier study had reported that among non-institutionalized elderly people, the spouse was often the only source of support (Shanas, 1979). However, marital problems do not seem to recede with age. Ruskin (1985) reported a study of sixty-seven patients over the age of sixty who had been referred to a geropsychiatric service at a teaching hospital. A quarter of these patients were facing family problems, and for them family therapy was the choice of treatment. Meunier (1994) noted that the most common cause for family therapy for elderly couples is the illness of a spouse. Any major change in the pattern of living can put marriages under strain.

However, it remains a fact that other than clinical reports on family therapy with elderly chronic pain patients, the extent of family problems in these families is a matter of speculation. Nevertheless, common sense dictates that marital and family problems must abound among elderly chronic pain sufferers, and if Mrs Thomas's case is an illustration of family issues, then it may be surmised that the problems are very complex, indeed.

THE BURDEN OF CARING

Mrs Thomas, in addition to coping with her own health problems, had the responsibility of caring for a husband who had Alzheimer's disease. Before we consider the literature that examines the pros and cons of one elderly person taking care of a sick partner, we shall briefly review the impact of her husband's behaviour on Mrs Thomas's health. It took two years from the time of the first signs of memory loss and confusion until his admission to a nursing home. Mr Thomas's behaviour became increasingly unpredictable and at times violent. The health consequences on the caregivers of an Alzheimer's patient have come under sustained examination in recent decades. We shall briefly review this literature of the past decade.

The concept of 'burden' is apt in describing the difficulties that caregivers experience in relation to Alzheimer's patients. The principal findings of studies on this topic, taken together, show that the caregivers are placed at considerable risk for psychological and physical problems (Bedard et al., 2001; Karla-wish et al., 2001; Mayer, 2001; Shanks-McElroy and Strobino, 2001; Tebb and Jivanjee, 2000).

The relationship between the stress of caregiving and physiological distress is a well-researched subject, and in relation to the stress of caregiving a recent study revealed that this stress can exact the ultimate price of death. Schulz and Scott (1999) analysed 400 older spouses who were caregivers and compared them with a control group without the caregiving responsibility. Among the caregivers, who found the task stressful, the death rate was 63 per cent higher over a four-year period than among the non-caregivers. Those who did not find the task stressful had only slightly higher death rates compared with controls. Most deaths were attributable to an existing condition, although 5 per cent of the mortalities had no apparent cause.

A review of 1,028 articles from 1986 to 1992 investigated the impact of chronic disease in the elderly on the physical and psychological health of the members' of the patient's family (Kriegsman, Penninx, and van Eijk, 1994). Alzheimer's disease was the most common condition reported. Both the psychological and physical health of the caregivers was adversely affected. The female spouses of elderly male patients were the most vulnerable, especially if they lacked social support.

A recent review confirmed that female caregivers were at greatest risk for psychiatric morbidity (Yee and Schulz, 2000). Vitaliano et al. (1996) examined the relationship between the psychological stress of caregiving and metabolic variables. Fasting insulin and glucose levels were assessed in two groups of non-diabetic subjects. One group comprised caregivers of Alzheimer's patients and the other gender-matched spouses of non-demented partners. The results showed that the caregivers of Alzheimer's patients had significantly higher insulin levels than controls over a period of fifteen to eighteen months. The conclusion was that relationship between care-giving and psychological and physiological distress exist both cross-sectionally and over time.

Cohen et al. (1990) investigated whether the stress of caregiving alters cellular immune response to acute psychological stressors. Subjects were women caring for a spouse with a progressive dementia and a matched control group without caregiving responsibility. The results suggested that although the stress of caregiving diminished cellular immune function, caregiving seemed to have little effect on cellular immune responses to or recovery from psychological challenges that were brief. Mrs Thomas developed breast cancer shortly after the her husband was placed in a nursing home. It would be erroneous to make any direct link between her trauma of caring, finally institutionalizing her husband, and the development of the carcinoma of her breast. Yet, the prospect that these life events and associated stress may have played some kind of a role does offer a tantalizing challenge.

Several studies have reported positive associations between caregiving of Alzheimer's patients and psychological and physical distress and disease (Cacioppo, Poehlmann, and Kiecolt-Glaser, et al., 1998; Kriegsman, Penninx, and van Eijk, 1994; Lieberman and Fisher, 1995; Pruchno et al., 1990; Pruchno and Potashnik, 1989). The role of personality and social supports in buffering spouses of Alzheimer's patients is highly significant. Monahan and Hooker (1995) reported that multivariate linear regression analyses of the effects of perceived social support, personality, and the gender of the caregiver explained 28 per cent of such variance, which was highly significant. It may be recalled that Mrs Thomas had little in the way of social support (other than the pain clinic), and clearly she felt victimized by her husband's illness. In fact, her only child was opposed to the institutionalization of his father. Precisely what effect these factors had on Mrs Thomas's overall health is difficult to determine. What may not be denied is that Mrs Thomas's level of anxiety and depression became markedly worse over a prolonged period.

Although the literature is equivocal about the negative health effects of caregiving, from a clinical point of view several aspects are noteworthy in relation to the case of Mrs Thomas.

She was indeed very anxious and depressed about her husband's predicament. The frequency of her visits to the clinic went up significantly during the period after his diagnosis, and remained high. She also complained of more pain and, as noted, she developed breast cancer. Mrs Thomas showed a remarkable lack of concern about the cancer. To her, this was one more problem, but certainly not as pressing as the others. The pain clinic became the central source of her social support system.

DEATH OF MRS THOMAS'S SON

Mrs Thomas's middle-aged son died suddenly and unexpectedly of a cerebral hemorrhage. Her relationship with her son had, at best, been conflictual. He was the only child, and from a very early age had formed a strong bond with his father. He was altogether unconvinced of his mother's ailments, and had expressed doubts to the pain clinic staff about her endless complaints of aches and pain. He viewed her as overly domineering. Over the years, Mrs Thomas had often expressed misgivings about her son to the pain clinic staff. Following her son's death, Mrs Thomas remained utterly convinced that his death had been preventable. She managed to convince the coroner's office to have a second look at the case.

The reason for this brief incursion into Mrs Thomas's relationship with the son is simply to point out one of the complications of an unexpected death, which is in itself a traumatic event. The guilt Mrs Thomas experienced over her son's death found expression in her belief that he should not have died. In short, her grieving process was coloured by the quality of her relationship with her son. Her son, who had been somewhat of a disappointment to her in life (in his choice of profession and his choice of spouse, among other things), assumed in death the qualities of a most cherished son. Grieving the sudden death of a grown-up child, where the relationship in life had been an unhappy one, is complicated. We briefly review some of the current literature discussing the pertinent clinical issues that may present.

The negative health and psychological consequences of losing an adult child are considerable. One study with direct relevance to Mrs Thomas's case showed how bereavement was complicated when the relationship with an adult deceased child was conflictual. Rubin and Schechter (1998) studied fifty college students and fifty adults in their fifties who had completed demographic and loss-response questionnaires. These subjects believed that the bereaved were particularly affected, first, when the deceased was an adult child, and, second, where the relationship with the deceased was conflictual. Fitzpatrick (1998) in his review indicated that health was adversely affected by stressful recent events, such as death of a child, and that elderly men were particularly disadvantaged, as they showed higher rates of psychological and physical disorders. DeVries et al. (1997) also reported that a decline in health follows on the death of an adult child. These studies paint a picture of considerable risk for an elderly parent. In Mrs Thomas's case, the most telling impact was, at least from a clinical point of view, on her psychological functioning. In addition to manifesting grief, she directed her anger at the medical profession for her son's untimely death. At the time of this writing, Mrs Thomas has regained a great deal of her composure, but remains in a state of increased hostility with her daughter-in-law, who is now involved with another man. Her search for her son's 'true' cause of death continues. Mr Thomas was not fully aware of his son's death, and occasionally asked about his whereabouts. He died shortly afterwards.

Treatment Issues

Mrs Thomas's pain problems were so completely overwhelmed by these events that the emphasis shifted from psychological management of her pain to managing her loss and grief. During this period, Mrs Thomas's involvement with her primary physician at the pain clinic became more frequent. However, as she stated on more than one occasion, she no longer knew where and how she was hurting, other than that her pain had become unbearable. Although universal, grief is nevertheless a complex phenomenon. Grief can render people incapacitated. Grief may also set a course that deviates from normal grief, which is usually from a few weeks' to a few months' duration. However, grief assumes considerable complexity when it becomes prolonged and shows no sign of resolution. This type of grief is described as abnormal or pathological grief and can be a precursor to psychiatric problems. Another type of abnormal grief is delayed grief, which is grief postponed, and restoring it is usually complicated. Some of the signs of prolonged grief are the following: *an inability to accept the death of a loved one; *persistence of intense grief; *attempts to communicate with the dead person; *persistence of physical symptoms such as loss of appetite, sleep disturbance, aches, and pain; and *in some patients, severe depression and even suicidal thoughts or actions.

Some or all of these symptoms may be evident in prolonged grief. Delayed grief is also problematic and complicated and tends to share similar symptoms to prolonged grief (Parkes, 1983). There is much discussion in contemporary literature on the necessary stages of grief that one has to travel through to arrive at satisfactory resolution. Bowlby (1980) identified four distinct and yet overlapping stages: (1) shock, associated with numbness and denial; (2) yearning and protest, as realization of the loss develops; (3) despair, accompanied by somatic and emotional upset and social withdrawal; and (4) gradual recovery, marked by increased well-being and acceptance of loss.

Treatment for Mrs Thomas. was very complex. Her pain picture was hugely complicated by her losses. No sooner had she begun to adjust to her new reality, even resuming some of her favourite activities, than her son died unexpectedly. She was completely numbed by this event. Slowly, she began to grieve.

Throughout all of this, the pain clinic remained central to Mrs Thomas's care. Grief therapy was the mainstay of her treatment. Grief therapy has come under much scrutiny, and the types of therapy are indeed wide-ranging, from catharsis to family-oriented to cognitive-behavioural to ego-oriented therapy

(Allumbaugh and Hoyt, 1999; Barbato and Irwin, 1992; Kissane et al., 1998; Malkinson, 1996; Mahiacek, 1992; Stroebe, Schut, and Stroebe, 1998; Neimeyer, 1999; Worden, 1991; However, a recent meta-analysis of outcome studies shows that any kind of grief therapy produces but small-to-moderate treatment effects (Allumbaugh and Hoyt, 1999). Client selection procedure was identified as an important variable affecting treatment outcome across studies. The value or necessity of grief work for adjustment to bereavement is an issue of some debate and is discussed in a subsequent chapter. Cultural variations in the concepts of loss and grief and the associated coping responses have been cited as a basis for reformulating interventions.

Therapeutic interventions for facilitating grieving in older adults have been proposed by Frank et al. (1997). In addition, the formulation and treatment of loss and grieving have been addressed from a developmental perspective, which identifies grief as a naturally occurring phenomenon in the intergenerational family cycle (Shapiro, 1994). Although loss and grief are integral to the experience of chronic pain, grief therapy has been neglected in the literature that evaluates treatment. Reed (1999) examined the efficacy of grief therapy for sixty-one adults with co-morbid chronic pain and depression. Subjects who received grief therapy reported less pain and depression and decreased use of psychotropic medications and fewer visits to mental health care providers relative to the control group receiving standard treatment. No treatment effects were found for use of pain medications or utilization of options for medical care.

Catharsis, an integral part of grief therapy, was the primary approach adopted in treating Mrs Thomas's grief. An environment was created for her where she could give free expression to all her memories about her deceased son. She could seek reassurance that her feelings of uncontrolled crying and other behaviours unfamiliar to her were normal, and that she was 'not going out of her head.' The key ingredients to recovery from bereavement are: (1) intellectual recognition and emotional explanation for the loss and (2) emotional acceptance.

Mrs Thomas had no problem in accepting the reality of her son's death. Nevertheless, she had considerable difficulty in accepting the cause of his death, in part, because when her son first started complaining of headaches, his symptoms had not been taken seriously. Mrs Thomas's failure to find adequate emotional explanation for her son's death was, at the very least, not without foundation. The final element in the grief process is emotional acceptance of the loss. In this respect, Mrs Thomas made very rapid progress in therapy. In fact, she had a good grasp of that horrible reality almost from the beginning, and over time she accepted her son's death. Her struggle was with the cause of his death. In every other respect, Mrs Thomas has returned to her normal level of functioning. She managed to overcome her acute state of grief, although still challenging the cause of her son's death. Her grieving was very much within the parameters of normal grief. Mrs Thomas's cancer remained confined. She was very resentful about not being able to see her grandchildren, but realized that she had little control over that situation. The pain clinic continued to fulfil a central role as a major source of support for Mrs Thomas.

Epilogue

Mrs Thomas's husband died of a chest infection in the nursing home. Upon his death, Mrs Thomas followed a normal course of grief, and she even had a sense of relief that he had been 'released' from his suffering. At the time of this writing, Mrs Thomas's involvement with the pain clinic is only nominal, and she is no longer receiving active psychological therapy.

IS THIS PAIN OR GRIEF? – MS. UNA

The case of Ms. Una is presented to show a relatively common complication of grief when grief is presented in the guise of somatic symptoms. Ms. Una was referred to the pain clinic with an unremitting complaint of back pain of three years' duration. The pain kept her confined to her apartment, and she spent most of her waking hours in a supine position. She clearly was not taking adequate care of herself. In spite of numerous investigations for her pain, all the findings were negative.

Ms. Una never married because she had 'never had the time.' She started her retail business early in life and also had her mother to look after. She was highly regarded in the business community and participated to the full in business activities. As she approached the age of sixty-five, Ms. Una decided to sell her business to have more leisure, and also to devote more time to her unwell mother. She had a married sister with whom she enjoyed a close relationship.

This patient's pain began in earnest some six months after her retirement. A year later, her mother died. Ms. Una was now without a purpose in life and on the verge of assuming the status of an invalid. When seen at the pain clinic, she was depressed and looked unkempt. Seeing her in that state made it hard to imagine that in the recent past she had been a success- ful business woman. Ms. Una expressed great uncertainty about her future. She also had serious doubts about the negative medi- cal findings and was convinced that she had a serious as yet undiagnosed ailment.

Analysis

Ms. Una's main purpose for selling her business, which she had devoted her entire adult life to building up, was to have more leisure time and more time take care of her ailing mother. Her mother died soon after Ms. Una sold her business. Thus, her principal motivation for retirement was lost. It is equally im- portant to appreciate that Ms. Una had no social life outside her business world. She did not have a single close friend. Her social life was very circumscribed, but for a married sister whom she saw occasionally.

The death of her mother, who had been elderly and frail, was not altogether unanticipated. Yet, this death emerged as a ma- jor contributory factor in the deteriorating health of our pa- tient. Her pain problems were idiopathic, and yet her increased somatization was more than a coincidence with her mother's death. Her mother's death removed just about the only reason Ms. Una had for selling her business. She suffered two great losses in terms of her identity: first, as a successful business-woman, and then as a daughter. Another critical question has to be the mourning the death of her mother. It is notable that when Ms. Una first arrived at our clinic, she was very focused on her pain and disability, and it took time and effort to put her story together. Somatization as a form of conflicted grief is well noted in the literature (Bonanno et al., 1995; Parkes and Weiss, 1983; Winokuer, 2000).

In retrospect, pain problems which had begun to worsen soon after retirement, took a serious turn for the worse, and Ms. Una's entire attention was diverted to her deteriorating health. Under those circumstances it would be reasonable to assume that she had failed to grieve in a timely way, and her grieving assumed some of the characteristics of abnormal grief discussed earlier in this chapter.

Treatment

The problems stated by Ms. Una included pain, as might be expected. The death of her mother, selling her business, and the ensuing loneliness were readily pointed out by this patient. Although she did not make any connection between her altered circumstances and pain, which very few patients do, Ms. Una was certainly cognizant of her isolation and sadness.

The targeted problems to be worked on with Ms. Una in-cluded the following: (1) she had failed to grieve her mother's death; (2) she was spending an extraordinary amount of time lying in bed; (3) she was not adequately taking care of herself; and (4) she was shunning all social contact.

All of Ms. Una's problems were clearly in the category of reactive emotional distress. She was a highly efficient business woman and homemaker. She enjoyed her life and before this had never had a day's illness. Now with things gone so wrong, Ms. Una was anxious to regain her health.

The contract with Ms. Una included six sessions over a two-month period. The goals of treatment were: (a) signs of acceptance of her mother's death and her own grief; (b) a measurable level of increased daily activity, (c) evidence of self-care, and (d) restoration of social contact. The tasks were carefully designed around each goal, and within the specified time she had not only achieved her goals, but surpassed them. Grief and loss were at the heart of her pain symptoms. Given the superb state of her premorbid abilities, it was hardly surprising that Ms. Una made a remarkable recovery.

CONCLUSION

This chapter has made an attempt to show that pain, chronic illness, and grief coexist in elderly people, probably more so than in any other age group. The simple and obvious reason for this is that old age is characterized by multiple losses. Full comprehension of these issues and their incorporation into the treatment plan for such a patient is imperative. Much has been written recently about 'ageism' which has prevented the elderly chronic pain sufferers from fully benefiting from the plethora of psychological interventions for pain management. There is evidence that when such treatments are made available, elderly patients seem to benefit a great deal. The fact, however, remains that elderly patients are somewhat rare in a pain clinic setting. This would suggest that mental health professionals working with geriatric patients in medical settings should begin to pay more attention to incorporating psychological and social methods for pain control.

8

Chronic Illness and Suicide:
The Ultimate Loss

Suicide among the chronically ill, although relatively infrequent, does occur. The reasons for suicide in this population are varied, but they tend to fall into two broad categories: (1) existential reasons and (2) clinical depression. In terms of existential reasons, recognition that one's quality of life is severely compromised through one's illness and disability, together with the acknowledgment that one is being a burden to others, makes suicide seem like a viable option to ending the misery. Clinical depression, as the literature review will show, is emerging as the single most powerful reason for suicide in this population. The topic of assisted suicide, however, is too complex and controversial to include in this discussion more than in this passing way. Yet, the very idea of assisted suicide is a reflection of the desperate state of these patients who seek such help.

In this chapter, first, we will present a brief overview of the current literature on (1) chronic illness and suicide, (2) cancer and suicide, and (3) chronic pain and suicide. Second, we shall present two cases of completed suicide in an effort to understand the underlying causes that may have contributed to the tragic and premature deaths of these individuals. Third, we shall present the case of a young woman with suicidal thoughts and intentions. A great deal of the literature on suicide in the medically ill examines the risk of suicide and depression, and this last case is a good illustration of how that literature may be applied.

CHRONIC ILLNESS AND SUICIDE

A point of note is that the literature on chronic illness and suicide is a mixed bag in the sense that it encompasses thoughts of suicide to attempted suicide to completed suicide. In a comprehensive review of the literature on the desire of the seriously chronically or terminally ill patients to hasten death, Mishara (1999) examined the presenting factors. These included patient characteristics, factors associated with chronic disease, depression, coping strategies, premorbid suicidability, and the desire to hasten death. Mishara claimed that depression as a factor in suicide could not be supported by empirical evidence. Depression, indeed, could be a direct physiological symptom of pathology associated with the disease. Furthermore, a depressive reaction could also be a side-effect of treatment for the illness. Many medications could cause depressive symptoms, and the prolonged use of high doses of some medications may result in a high risk of developing a depressive reaction. Mishara (1999) concluded that 'many disabilities and physical illnesses also precipitate changes in social interactions and participation in daily life. The limitations caused by these diseases may result in social isolation, loss of close relationships with friends, co-workers, and a general feeling of worthlessness. These social effects of the illness, rather than the illness or disability itself, may be the determining factors related to suicidal behaviour.' Yet, surprisingly, Mishara's literature review failed to substantiate this perspective with evidence.

There is considerable evidence suggesting that persons with chronic illness have a higher rate of suicide (Lewis, 2001). Feelings of hopelessness, together with poor quality of life, tend to contribute to suicidal behaviour. Ernst (1997) conducted an extensive literature review of the epidemiology of depression and suicide in late life. Physical illness was commonly associated with minor depression. Yet, risk factors such as decline in self-perceived health, somatic symptoms, functional impairment, serious objective health problems, and loss of independence were readily observed in the older population. Ernst reviewed a survey of literature on suicide attempts in old age. Physical illness, living alone, loneliness, and disturbed intimate relationships emerged as frequently occurring factors. The major conclusion was that late onset depression connected with brain dysfunction, a slow course, and often an imperfect recovery were the main factors accounting for the prevalence of depression and suicide in late life. In addition, however, factors such as somatic illness, pain and organic brain syndromes rather than major depression and dysthymia made an older person more vulnerable to depressive symptoms and even suicide.

In a comprehensive study of factors associated with suicidal ideation in adults, which made it somewhat of an exceptional study, Vilhjalmsson and associates (1998) used data from a health survey of 825 adult residents in the city of Reykjavik, Iceland. Multiple chronic conditions, frequent alcohol use, and various forms of distress, which included pain, were related to thoughts of suicide. In addition, low self-esteem and a low sense of mastery (both relatively commonly observed in people who are chronically ill) were associated with suicidal ideation. In short, chronic illness, pain in conjunction with low self-esteem and loss of mastery created an optimum environment in which people might consider suicide. These authors concluded that 'suicide ideation in adults finds that people in highly stressful domestic, financial, and particularly legal circumstances, who experience extensive physical health problems and who perceive their lives as stressful are more likely to contemplate suicide.' It is noteworthy that many of the same problems can also be the direct consequence of a serious or chronic physical illness. This will become evident in the first case we shall discuss in this chapter. Confirmation of the conclusion was found in a major epidemiological study on completed suicide among elderly people in China, where common causes of suicide were found to be chronic illness and family and psychological problems (Xu et al., 2000).

The quality-of-life issue was examined in a study of adolescents with epilepsy by Andelman (2000). For children with epilepsy, the quality of life was closely related to depression, anxiety, and locus of control. These children experienced more depression (internalizing behaviour problems) and suicide attempts compared with those with chronic illness.

In a comprehensive study of emotional distress and suicidal ideation among 3,129 adolescents aged fourteen to nineteen years, Suris and associates (1996) indexed a group of 162 children among four chronic conditions: asthma, diabetes, seizure, and cancer. No significant differences in emotional distress or suicidal ideation emerged between those four groups of patients. Comparison with the control group of 865 subjects revealed that chronic illnesses was associated with substantive emotional distress and thoughts of suicide in teenage girls. Over 23 per cent of the adolescent girls in this study who had a chronic illness had suicidal thoughts compared with 8.9 per cent of the female subjects without chronic illness. One in every four females and one in every six males reported that they had had thoughts of suicide. These rates for youths with chronic conditions were substantially higher than for the entire sample of adolescents. This study provides convincing evidence that thoughts of suicide are relatively common in young people with chronic conditions.

This body of rather divergent studies suggests that social and psychological factors provide major reasons for suicide. Almost all the studies reviewed here show the primacy of social factors, rather than mental illness in general and depression in particular, as determinants of suicidal thoughts and behaviour. One important observation is that the significance of social factors in suicide seems to cut across age groups, from adolescence to the elderly, and across a multitude of medical conditions. Nevertheless, this review is but cursory and not too many hard and fast conclusions should be drawn from it.

CANCER AND SUICIDE

Hughes and Kleepsies (2001) noted that certain medical conditions are recognized for carrying a higher risk for suicide than others, or none. In this category of conditions, brain cancer was recognized as one such disease. In general terms, the literature on cancer and suicide falls into two categories. The first category demonstrates that most of the patients with cancer who attempt, or commit, suicide tend to manifest a measurable level of depression. Yet, in an in-depth analysis of five cancer patients who committed suicide, fear of losing autonomy and of being a burden to others emerged among an assortment of psychological and personality factors as the most powerful reasons for these completed suicides (Filiberti et al., 2001). Some of the other critical factors that may have contributed to the suicides were the following: functional and physical impairments, fear of suffering, uncontrolled pain, awareness of impending death, and mild-to-moderate depression. These five individuals who committed suicide had held managerial positions. They all had strong characters. Another feature of these patients was that four of them were married with children, while one was single. Four of these patients were in their sixties and seventies, while the fifth was but fifty years old.

The second category describes patients who want to end their life for social and existential reasons and who seek medically assisted suicide. The very topic of medically assisted suicide is fraught with medical, legal, social, religious, and ethical controversies, and for those reasons falls outside the scope of this work. Suffice to say that there now exists a significant body of literature on this topic.

The rate of diagnosed depression in cancer patients ranges from a low of 3.7 per cent to an astonishing 58 per cent. Lynch (1995) further noted that a review of the literature established that of hospitalized cancer patients with substantial physical impairment, 25 per cent suffered from 'clinically important' depression. In a study of 100 consecutive cancer patients (twenty-eight to eighty-six years of age) several depression scales were used to measure depression and suicidability (Ciaramella and Poli, 2001). Using the Structured Clinical Interview for DSM-III-R established the rate of depression at 29 per cent in this population. However, using the Hamilton Depression Rating Scale, showed that 49 per cent of the subjects were depressed. Age and sex were non-significant factors in predicting depression. Both scales identified suicide ideation. Patients who were found to be depressed on both scales also had more metastasis and pain, suggesting that the severity of the disease had a major influence in the presentation of depression.

However, an earlier study of sixty cancer patients who had completed suicide, showed that 80 per cent of them had given evidence of prior depressive syndromes (Henriksson et al., 1995). In a matched group of non-cancer suicides the rate of depression was 82 per cent. This suggests that depression in cancer-related suicide is almost identical to non-cancer suicides, and raises critical questions about the exact role that cancer itself may play as a determinant of the suicide in the case of cancer patients, or the extent to which cancer and associated suffering contribute to depression and suicide. The major conclusion of Henricksson et al.'s study was that mental illness was the major factor behind suicides in patients, with or without cancer. However, for cancer suicides, alcoholism and psychotic disorders were less common. In defence of their finding, these authors noted that DSM-III criteria were stringently applied, symptoms that might have been directly related to the disease excluded (an extremely difficult task), and their decision to err on the side of caution might have resulted in underestimation of some mental disorders. They also noted that 'suicide in good mental health is a rare event, even among victims who have suffered from malignant disease.' One intriguing factor that was not addressed in this study was the reason(s) behind suicide of those patients who were not depressed. In fact, the authors claimed that their findings did not support the rationality of cancer suicide.

A relationship between level of depression and suicide 'tendency' was noted in a study of thirty newly diagnosed cancer patients, fifty-one cancer patients who were receiving adjuvant chemotherapy, and thirty-three cancer patients with recurrence who were receiving chemotherapy (Gilbar and Eden, 2000–1). The Israeli Index of Potential Suicide (IIPS) was used to measure suicidability. Contrary to the hypothesis that cancer patients with recurrence had more tendencies toward suicide, depression, and hopelessness, no statistically significant differences emerged between the three groups. Overall, these findings showed a moderately significant correlation between suicidal tendency and depression in these cancer patients. An intriguing finding was an absence of any relationship between hopelessness as measured using the Beck Hopelessness Scale (BHS) and suicide tendency. Since hopelessness is common among depressed patients, this absence of any association defies common sense. One plausible explanation for this curious finding, according to the authors, was to be found in different instructions and different psychometric properties of the depression scales. The Beck Depression Inventory (BDI) was designed to measure depression in psychiatric patients (although it has been extensively used with the chronic pain population), while the symptoms of depression in cancer patients could be a response to the threat to life caused by the diagnosis in a normal population. Unlike the authors of the previous study, Gilbar and Eden did not ascribe suicidal tendencies to psychiatric disorders.

In an earlier population-based study in Stockholm County (Sweden), undertaken between 1975 and 1985, 59,845 cancer patients were identified (Allebeck and Bolund, 1991). Of these, 144 completed and another 196 attempted suicide in the follow-up period. First and foremost, unlike the study by Gilbar and Eden, this study found that presence of cancer did significantly add to the risk of completed suicides. The rate of suicide attempts was only moderately higher in cancer patients than in the general population. Allebeck and Bolund raised questions about depression and emotional distress among cancer patients and their role in suicides. The progression of cancer, level of social and physical impairment, and the frequent losses experienced by these patients constituted important sources of their depression and emotional distress. For these reasons, patients with advanced stages of cancer or rapidly progressing cancer were strongly associated with suicide rates. Psychosocial factors rather than psychiatric disorders were found to be dominant as determinants of suicide in cancer patients.

Akechi et al. (2001) examined differences in the background among of cancer patients with major depression, with and without suicidal ideation. They observed that uncontrolled pain, advanced illness, loss of control, and hopelessness were all recognized as factors making people vulnerable to suicide. The precise role of depression in suicidability in cancer patients was the focus of this study. In a group of 1,721 patients, 220 (12.8 per cent) had major depression and of these, 113 had reported thoughts of suicide. Two factors, namely, poor physical functioning and severe depression emerged as significant risk factors. Cancer patients with major depression who were not engaged in full- or part-time employment, who had a poor record of job performance, and who had more severe depression were potentially at risk for suicide and needed and required intensive monitoring to prevent suicide. This is a curious finding, as patients with cancer who were also depressed were not very likely to perform well in their jobs. Physical functioning as well as depression were identified as important risk factors for suicide. Implicit in this finding is the inextricable relationship between the level of disability and the degree of depression.

The prevailing wisdom supported by data seems to indicate that cancer increases the risk for suicide. Nevertheless, in a study of depression and suicide in people over the age of sixty, Lawrence and associates (2000) provided data to the contrary. In a retrospective review of suicide attempts and suicides between 1980 and 1995 in Western Australia, one relevant finding for this discussion was the discovery of an inverse association between the diagnosis of cancer among elderly mental health patients and suicide. Elderly patients with cancer were 3.6 times less likely to commit suicide. These authors acknowledged that their finding was contrary to others and attributed the differences to divergent study populations. They speculated that the diagnosis of cancer in patients with a history of mental illness placed them under greater medical surveillance, thus providing greater social and psychological supports and thus reducing the risk of suicide.

This body of literature is truly challenging because the conclusions of the various individual studies are so much at variance with each other. It seems that cancer alone is not a sufficient reason for suicide (Henriksson et al., 1995). Only major depression accounts for suicide, claims one study. In contrast, the Swedish study concluded that cancer significantly added to the risk of suicide (Allebeck and Bolund, 1991). On the surface, these differences appear to be irreconcilable until we address the issues raised by Mishara (1999) in his review that depression could very well be related in simple as well as in complex ways with illness.

CHRONIC PAIN AND SUICIDE

This body of literature is limited. In a survey of 204 patients with chronic but non-malignant pain, with an average of 9.5 years duration, only 50 per cent reported inadequate pain relief (Hitchcock, Ferrell, and McCaffery, 1994). The respondents identified multiple losses such as the inability to work or carry out household chores, limitations of activities, and fatigue as the worst problems resulting from their pain. Hitchcock et al. noted that 'perhaps the most alarming is the observation that, in spite of their substantial social and financial resources, 50% of subjects had considered suicide.' This illustrates the enormous impact of chronic pain, and adds to the growing evidence that chronic pain can be life-threatening.

Amir and associates (2000) examined suicide risk, among other factors, in a group of women with fibromyalgia. Their key finding was that women who had chronic pain, not only fibromyalgia, but also with chronic lower back pain and rheumatoid arthritis, were more likely than not to use an avoidant coping style, more state anger, and more turn anger inward, in addition to being at greater risk for suicide. However, these authors urged caution in interpreting the suicide data since they had performed multiple comparisons, and no individual group showed any significant difference compared with normal women.

Chronic pain patients, who had experienced childhood abuse, were found to show a high risk for suicide. In an investigation of 379 adult patients, Barron (1997) showed that 42 per cent reported some form of abuse during their growing up years. Overall, the abused group made greater use of medical and mental health services, made more suicide attempts, and had elevated scores on affective and sensory pain rating scales, suggesting psychological distress.

Fisher and his colleagues (2001) confirmed Hitchcock et al.'s concern that the rates of completed suicides are higher in the chronic pain population than in the general population. They investigated 200 chronic pain subjects in an in-patient rehabilitation unit. Thirteen of these individuals (6.5 per cent) reported thoughts of suicide using the Beck Depression Inventory. These thirteen individuals were compared with similarly depressed, non-suicidal individuals and a matched group of non-depressed individuals. The findings were complex. A history of substance abuse was higher in both depressed groups. The depressed groups did not differ from each other on any of the measures of the pain experience. Depression, and not suicidal status, consistently predicted the level of functioning. One curious finding was that physical pain alone did not predict a desire to die. The other point of note was that not one patient expressed suicidal intent without presenting clinically significant symptoms of depression. Fisher and colleagues proposed that future studies should examine genetic, biological, psychological, and social factors that could be protective factors for suicidal intent, suicide attempts, or completed suicides.

While the previous studies dealt with suicidal thoughts and attempts, Kewman and Tate (1998) reported a case study involving a man with a spinal cord injury who committed suicide. He was thirty-three years old. This study investigated in depth the factors that could have contributed to this man's suicide. Among other factors, poor social adjustment, poor body image, unremitting chronic pain, and a prolonged history of abuse of prescription drugs were found as explanatory factors for his premature death. Just a day before his suicide, he had consulted a psychologist who evidently had told him that he would have to learn to live with his pain. According to this man's wife, the patient was devastated with that assessment. The next day he killed himself. It would be erroneous to attribute his suicide solely to the conversation with the psychologist. Nevertheless, confirmation that he would have to live with the reality of pain and disability was unacceptable to this patient. Such an individual case study is of some import as it is an attempt to look beyond psychiatric disorder(s) explanations for suicide. It would be reasonable to assume that given his circumstances, this man probably would have been found to be depressed, and his suicide attributed to his psychiatric state, but the underlying causes for his depression may have been overlooked.

The complex nature of the relationship between chronic pain and depression has been the topic of much debate for the past several decades. There is now a general acceptance of two facts: (1) A proportion of chronic pain sufferers also suffer from clinical depression. (2) The misfortune that emanates from chronic pain conditions also contributes to the development of depressive symptoms. In other words, social factors are critically important to fully appreciate the psychological state of chronic pain sufferers.

The causes precipitating suicidal thoughts, attempts, and completed suicide for medically ill patients are complex at best. As our brief look at the literature shows, while some researchers show a very high level of confidence in claiming a relationship between depression and suicide, the work of others points in the opposite direction. This observation is true of all three patient populations discussed in this review.

Summary

In general terms, the literature on illness and suicide points in the direction of a robust relationship between the level of depression and suicide. Although there is acknowledgment that social and psychological factors play a role in suicide in medically ill patients, studies fall short in demonstrating their significance compared with clinical or major depression.

A most problematic issue that remains is the propensity of disease and disability to engender depression. Losses are common in the populations described above. Major changes in roles and identities of individual patients present daily challenges. Medication and other types of medical intervention are also capable of producing depression or depressive symptoms. Depression is not that infrequently an integral part of many diseases. Given this level of complexity, high levels of depression seem likely. On the other hand, in the population of patients who have chronic illness or disability the presence of even a significant level of depression is not sufficient to produce suicidal intent or attempts. Perhaps, critical factors such as social supports, personality, and demographic factors play more obvious roles than we have up to now thought was the case in determining the suicidal potential of medically ill patients.

A CASE OF EMASCULATION? — MR JAMES

Mr James (see Chapter 3) not long after immigrating to Canada, had realized his dream of finding a good job, marrying, and having three children. He was very settled when he incurred a work-related injury involving his right hip and leg. Mr James was expected to recover in a short time, and was placed on workers' compensation. But instead of improving, his condition proceeded to deteriorate, and he embarked on a journey to find a medical cure for his pain and for his disability. His search for cure proved futile. As a result, Mr James became increasingly hostile towards the medical profession.

Mr James, as it turned out, was not able to return to work. He lost his job, and his workers' compensation was discontinued. Thus, began a long and futile battle with the Workers' Compensation Board. Being confined to his house gradually turned Mr James into, according to his children, a tyrant. He had been a good partner, father and provider, but now he neglected his responsibilities to his family, lost interest in sex, and consumed large doses of prescription tranquillizers and narcotic analgesics to control his pain. Mr James's behaviour had become erratic. He would undertake household projects that he could not possibly finish. This had the double effect of becoming a further challenge to his 'manhood' and, second, it led him to blame his children for what he perceived to be their callous attitude towards his predicament. They, on the other hand, felt that there was no way of pleasing him.

Mr James was a traditional man with deeply held values about gender roles. He was authoritarian with rather rigid views about masculine roles. Many of his valued roles were lost as a result of his accident and ensuing pain and disability, together with his deteriorated financial state due to both losing his job and losing workers' compensation benefits. He was unable to provide for his family, his libido had vanished, and he became unsure about his place in the family. Until his job loss, he was very definitely the head of the family.

This man's condition produced profound changes in his family. His wife had to assume virtually all the responsibilities of keeping the family together, meeting the challenges of ever increasing financial hardship, and trying to keep her husband appeased. Their three children were having problems. John had more or less disappeared from the domestic scene. Mary was depressed, and Marc was now into hard drugs. Until his job loss, Mr James had been a caring father who had spent many hours playing with his children when they were younger, and despite his strict ways, the children used to feel close to him.

When first seen at our pain clinic, the most obvious aspect of Mr James's behaviour was his anger – not only with the medical system, but virtually with every system he had ever had to interact with. It was easy to detect in his utterances that he almost believed there was a kind of conspiracy against him. He had always been a hard-working man. He was at a loss in trying to figure out what it was that he had done to deserve the scorn of his doctors, who seemed always underestimated his pain and suffering, and the Workers' Compensation Board that deprived him of his livelihood? Being forced onto welfare was almost the last straw for this man.

Mr James showed many signs and symptoms of abnormal illness behaviour, the most prominent of which was his conviction that his pain was somatic, and also his complete rejection of any possibility of psychological explanation for his pain and suffering. Second, there was evidence of affective disturbance. He was more angry than sad, and yet just underneath his overt anger was a profound sense of failure. Nevertheless he refused psychiatric consultation.

With his family and personal life apparently beyond redemption, Mr James became active in an organization for chronic pain patients. He organized meetings with the Workers' Compensation Board as well as with representatives of various provincial ministers. He became very successful in mobilizing many members of the organization in working for changes in the legislation governing workers' compensation. This phase lasted some nine or ten months, at the end of which time Mr James disappeared from the scene, as far as our clinic was concerned. We next heard of him after his suicide. Mr James killed himself with an overdose of tranquillizers and narcotic analgesics. The coroner's verdict was that Mr James had taken his own life. He was forty-five years old.

Analysis

The key question is, Why did Mr James kill himself? Any and all answers to this question are likely to be speculative. He did not leave a suicide note. Nevertheless, we shall attempt to understand Mr James's predicament in terms of his personal, family, and medico-social perspectives. He refused any ongoing psychotherapeutic endeavour, yet every now and again he would call his therapist at our clinic for a chat. The therapist met with the family as a whole on five occasions, and there was some evidence of improvement in the overall functioning of this family.

The fundamental problems remained, however. These were Mr James's health and his search for justice remained. Mr James's personal history strongly supported his belief that he had the primary responsibility for his family, and his role as the head of this family remained unquestioned by him. He had very fixed notions of his responsibilities. He had been the family's only provider and his wife never worked outside their home.

This was a father with an authoritarian style, and primary disciplinarian of his children. He was stern and held very high expectations of them. Yet, the children reported that Mr James was kind and totally committed to their well-being. He used to be a kind husband and the marriage had been relatively free of strife. In other words, Mr James's authoritarianism was rooted in both his belief that he was the sole head of the household and his equally rigid notion of masculinity. His accident and rapid deterioration into chronic disability deprived him his core identity roles, that of a man in the most traditional sense, a caring parent, and a husband. Each of these roles were put in jeopardy.

When the above facts are considered together with the rapid disintegration of the family's customary alignment, Mr James's profound sense of failure and desperation become apparent. As already noted, his children, each of whom had functioned normally and successfully prior to his accident, developed psychological and behavioural problems. Mr James held himself to be completely responsible for this state of affairs. His inability to alter the situation made him feel only more desperate. A great gulf developed between Mr James and his children. There were signs of strife in their marriage, as Mrs James was finding the added responsibilities hard to carry, and at times she would fail to be as supportive towards her husband as she had customarily been.

On the medical front, Mr James's feelings could only be described as those of utter hopelessness mixed with anger. He felt severely diminished as a human being by the medical establishment because it would not take his medical problems seriously and, more importantly, would not find a cure. These feelings were compounded by his interminable and, in the end, unwinnable battle with the Workers' Compensation Board. Being on welfare was very demeaning to him and left him feeling deeply humiliated.

The losses incurred by Mr James were significant. Loss of his employment, his health, his multiple family roles, and in his eyes, his very manhood were all contributory factors towards his suicide. One plausible explanation for his suicide may be found in his acutely developed idea of what it meant to be a man, and the steadfastness with which he hung on to this idea and all the responsibilities that went with it. Nothing short of a restoration of his pre-morbid health and lifestyle was going to be acceptable to Mr James. In the end he paid the ultimate price for his perceived failure to live up to his own definition of self.

Given his new reality, Mr James had to redefine himself. He was unable or, more probably, unwilling to redefine his identity to his satisfaction, and the identity that was thrust upon him he found unacceptable. Would Mr James have fared better had he agreed to a psychiatric assessment? Hopelessness and loss of self-esteem were at the heart of his despair, and clinical depression is not the sole cause for such psychological predicaments. Whether Mr James was suffering from clinical depression at the time of his suicide will never be known for certain.

Poor physical health, unresolved legal problems, financial problems, perception of life as very stressful, and poor interpersonal relationships were identified as reasons for suicide in an Icelandic study undertaken by Vilhjalmsson et al. (1998). Chronic rather than acute pain has also been associated with suicide (Bengesser, 1998). Sadly, Mr James was burdened with the presence of all these issues.

AN ANGRY, IMPULSIVE MAN: MR VINCE

Mr Vince presented with a history of mixed headaches that dated back to his adolescence. He was referred to our pain clinic because his headaches were getting worse. This was causing him to miss more and more time at work. Mr Vince worked as a labourer. In addition, his behaviour at the time we first saw him was becoming a concern at home. Frequently, he would lose his temper, and as this situation progressed, his children as well as his wife were becoming afraid of him.

Mr Vince described a history of impulsivity and poor self-control, which he attributed to having had his own way as a child with his parents. Although his parents had been very strict, when he had a headache they assumed all the characteristics of completely indulgent parents. Mr Vince confessed that, early in life, he had learned to use his headaches to get his own way. This pattern of behaviour spilled over into his marriage. He had a 'macho' sense of himself and attempted to dominate his wife and children in every conceivable way. Meanwhile, he had also managed to make a total mess of the family finances, until his wife had come to his rescue. Mr Vince felt slighted by his wife's evident success with money, and found novel ways of sabotaging her attempts to maintain some kind of order and equanimity in this family. It was only through Mrs Vince's determined efforts that the family's basic instrumental needs continued to be met. But the emotional issues remained unaddressed. When this couple and their children were seen for the first time at our clinic, the family was on the verge of disintegration.

Mr Vince presented perhaps an extreme form of rigid behaviour. As a chronic sufferer of headaches, for his comfort he demanded complete compliance with his rules, not only from his young children, but also from his wife. Failure to comply with his wishes resulted in some form of punishment as far as the children were concerned, and in serious acrimony between Mr Vince and his wife. When this couple arrived for their initial marital assessment, it was obvious that Mrs Vince was afraid of her husband. She confessed that in spite of their long years of marriage, she lived in fear of being hit by him. Although he had never actually physically abused her, he had often engaged in terrible verbal abuse. In addition, often he would refuse to talk to her for prolonged periods of time. Mrs Vince said the whole family lived as if they were 'walking on eggshells.' But Mr Vince's behaviour had a very interesting twist. Mr Vince became the model of a tolerant and understanding father and husband in those periods when he had a headache.

Mr Vince was treated with a combination of marital therapy, cognitive-behavioural therapy (CBT), and antidepressant and analgesic medications. He made remarkable progress. He became virtually pain free, and his behaviour moderated to the point that his wife was able to report that their marriage had never been better. During this phase Mr Vince had an automobile accident in which he sustained a back injury. There was no apparent reason to believe that he would not recover from this setback. One immediate consequence of the accident was Mr Vince's inability to work, which forced him to go on sickness benefits. His reaction to this development was overwhelming. Mr Vince's anger became almost unmanageable and completely impervious to reason. Vociferously, he would insist repeatedly that he was the unluckiest man on earth and that nothing ever went his way. He said he was born to be a loser. For a while Mr Vince withdrew from the pain clinic. He did come back, showing signs of improvement. On his last visit to the clinic, Mr Vince seemed cheerful. He had talked about returning to work. But on the way home from our clinic, Mr Vince jumped from a bridge into a river and drowned. He was in his early fifties.

Analysis

Understanding Mr Vince's suicide is not easy. He killed himself at a time when his situation was improving, and he was getting closer to returning to work. His domestic situation, too, had become better, and was somewhat more stabilized from what it was immediately following his car accident.

Was Mr Vince depressed? Could his personality account for his behaviour? What were his social circumstances that might shed some light on his decision to kill himself? Answers to all these questions do not add up to a satisfactory explanation for this suicide. Unquestionably Mr Vince was impulsive. Also, he believed that there was some kind of conspiracy operating to make his life miserable. No one, including his wife and children, seemed on his side to him. He saw himself as alone and unloved. Yet, Mr Vince had made significant gains in therapy. Then came his car accident. This was at a time when he was just beginning to gain some mastery over his headaches and the situation his family was in. The accident became further proof to him of his incurable ill fortune. When Mr Vince left the clinic that morning to go home, he gave no indication that committing suicide was on his mind. Just when he was starting to feel better again, Mr Vince killed himself. Perhaps he jumped into the river on impulse. At best, this is only a conjecture.

Perhaps, Mr Vince's conviction that he was put upon this earth only to experience constant pain and misery was at the root of this suicide. This, too, is a plausible explanation. Many depressed patients commit suicide – precisely not when in the depths of their depression, but as they begin to recover. Mr Vince was unquestionably getting better, but getting better for him might not have been such a positive prospect. It would have meant returning to his way of life which seemed to him to be full of interminable deep personal and interpersonal strife. The real reason for his suicide will unlikely ever be discovered. The literature discussed here sheds very little light on the reasons in explanation of a case like Mr Vince's suicide.

A CLEAR CASE OF DEPRESSION? – MRS WARNER

Mrs Warner was seen at our pain clinic three years after being involved in a rather unusual accident. She had been a passenger in a bus when it had come to a sudden stop. This caused her to lurch forward, and in doing so she injured both her knees and her right shoulder. Over a period of two months her shoulder pain worsened to the point that she became unable to continue at her job which involved manual labour at a furniture-making factory. Extensive radiological, neurological, and orthopaedic investigations failed to account for the loss of function and pain in her right shoulder.

Mrs Warner had a terrible history. She was sexually abused from the age of seven to nine years by a schoolteacher. This teacher threatened her with her life if she was to say anything about it to anyone. Furthermore, she was molested by her two older brothers during this same period. She tried to tell her mother about the brothers, but her mother would not believe her. When Mrs Warner was in Grade 11, the whole matter came to a head. For reasons that she could not explain, she became very depressed and would cry frequently, even in the class-room. She was seen by a school counsellor and, for the first time, was able to tell her story and be taken seriously. Her parents were brought into the picture, and in due course they came to accept that they had been negligent in not giving any credence to their daughter's story. The healing process had begun.

Mrs Warner completed high school, found a secure job, and married a very decent man, who man was of a different ethnic origin. Her family had serious objections to the marriage, and persisted in expressing them throughout the first four years of her married life. During that time, Mrs Warner had very limited contact with her family. She did not mind this state of affairs because she was very happy in her marriage and had no doubts about having married the right man. The only thing missing in her life was a child. This couple had virtually given up all hope of ever becoming parents, when soon after her accident she became pregnant. The pregnancy was a very difficult one, and the baby was born several weeks prematurely, weighing just over four pounds. Mrs Warner blamed herself for this. To make matters worse, she found it very hard to take care of the baby because of her virtually immobile right arm. On three separate occasions the baby had slipped out of her arms and fallen. Fortunately, on all three occasions the baby was left unharmed. From the very birth of her child, Mrs Warner adopted a view of herself as an inadequate mother. These feelings were signifi-cantly accentuated by the falls the baby endured and the wors-ening of her disability. At the time that Mrs Warner presented at our clinic, her baby is a thriving little girl twenty-one months of age. Mrs Warner had homecare to help her with household chores and the care of the baby.

There was an additional problem encountered by this pa-tient. Following the accident, Mrs Warner started receiving fi-nancial benefits from the automobile insurance company (which is publicly owned). Apparently, for purposes of checking the

veracity of her disability, she was tailed by an insurance investigator, so she believed. This became a source of enormous
distress for her, and revived the feelings of helplessness that
she had experienced in her childhood during the years she was
being abused. Eventually, she reported this matter to the po-
lice. She also confronted the insurance people. It took some
time before this situation was resolved.

When seen for psychosocial evaluation at the pain clinic, Mrs
Warner was clearly distraught. She cried through most of the
session and much of what she said focused on her failure as a
mother. In the course of routine mental status examination,
she revealed, in the midst of very loud crying, that she had
been giving a lot of thought to killing herself. As recently as the
week before, she had locked herself in the bedroom to swallow
a handful of 'pills.' But then she had thought about the baby
and her husband and become unable to go through with it. The
assessment of Mrs Warner's mental state showed persistently
low mood, lack of energy, lack of any sense of enjoyment, and
an almost a total loss of libido. She was sleeping only two to
three hours per night. Her appetite was compromised, although
there was no weight loss. Mrs Warner acknowledged that she
was having frequent crying spells, but never in front of other
people. She had not confided to her husband that she was having thoughts of suicide. Another critical aspect of her psychological state was her pervasive guilt about dropping the baby.
The family's history for depression was negative.

Analysis

The question in the case of Mrs Warner is the extent to which
her history of abuse complicates the clinical picture. That there
is a complex and intriguing relationship between abuse and
chronic pain has received limited empirical support. Childhood
abuse has been shown to have a strong association with a variety of psychiatric disorders, among them depression.

Mrs Warner had given ample evidence of tremendous resiliency. She had finished high school, obtained steady employment, and married the man she loved against the wishes of her

family. In other words, with the help of school counsellors and through her own resiliency, Mrs Warner had overcome or had come to terms with what can only be described as horrible childhood experiences.

The accident and subsequent and worsening disability created a new situation of jeopardy for the patient. Being followed by an investigator revived some of her past terror. Beyond that, Mrs Warner became ever more disabled and her self-esteem was greatly insulted. It is impossible to get an approximate measure of the impact of childhood abuse on Mrs Warner's present situation, other than to say the obvious that she had been made enormously helpless and vulnerable. Her inability to take care of her baby was almost beyond Mrs Warner's comprehension. In these circumstances, it would not be unusual for a woman to develop significant level of depression and suicidal ideation.

CONCLUSION

The central clinical issue in this discussion has to be effective case findings and measures targeting the prevention of suicide. Evidence suggests that chronic and painful illnesses do contribute to the risk for suicide. The role of major depression leading to suicidal behaviour in patients with a chronic medical condition, although somewhat imprecise, should not and cannot be underestimated. From a clinical perspective, an argument can certainly be made that diagnosis of depression and appropriate intervention measures should be undertaken even with patients who may only be marginally depressed. This is a better option than missing significant depression that may lead to suicide. In this context it is important to recognize any pre-existing psychopathology, as well as any previous history of self-destructive behaviour associated with certain kind of personalities, together with any family history of depression and suicide.

Part of the problem in this debate is the 'either/or' proposition. Are we looking at a case of clinical depression leading to suicide? Or, is suicide a conscious decision made by a mentally sound individual who has assessed her situation as being one of hopelessness and has chosen suicide? The entire discussion of assisted suicide is predicated on ensuring that even very ill patients may be of sound mind and entirely capable of making a choice for suicide.

The clinical issue that remains important, however, is the need to recognize the risk factors for suicide in the population of patients who have a chronic medical illness. Proper psychiatric and psychosocial assessment can certainly minimize the risk for suicide, although never completely eliminate it. Mrs Warner's case is such an example. The previous two cases are of special interest because suicidal risks for those two patients were never seriously even considered. On reflection, it may be said that, given Mr James's personal and cultural beliefs, such as what it meant to him to be a man, which meant he lost his core identity, he was a patient at risk for suicide. This particular loss from his point of view was irretrievable, and life without his capacity to be a 'man' was, for him, not worth living.

Mr Vince poses an even greater challenge to our understanding. His impulsivity and general lack of control should be construed as risk factors for suicide. The way he killed himself very much suggests that, in all probability, his suicide was an act of impulse. Perhaps, the lesson in working with a patient who has a chronic medical illness is to routinely conduct an assessment of mental status, a thorough family history of depression and suicide, and continually observe the level despondency and hopelessness. There appears to be almost an 'organic' link between depression and hopelessness.

Lynch (1995), in her excellent review, noted that 86 per cent of suicides who were cancer patients occurred in the terminal phase. She concluded that the single most important issue related to suicidal vulnerability was a sense of loss of control or helplessness. This included not only loss of physical control, but even more distressing, the sense of losing control of one's mind. Perhaps, both our patients were overwhelmed by a feeling of having lost control over their lives.

9

Grief Therapy

Much of the literature on grief therapy concerns death and dying, as was discussed in an earlier chapter (see Chapter 7). Coming to terms with one's own death, and working through the process of bereavement after the death of a loved one are the heart and soul of the published material on grief therapy. The overwhelming majority of people come to terms with the grief following the death of someone they have been close to without the benefit of psychotherapy. Grief therapy, which is integral to psychotherapy, becomes necessary only where there are indications that the grieving process has deviated from the usual and generally predictable course. At its simplest, grief therapy creates an opportunity for the bereaved to engage in catharsis, which is a process of letting go by saying everything that there is to say about the deceased. The therapeutic process itself has the two following goals: (1) recognition of the loss, that is, overcoming denial and, (2) arriving at acceptance.

It is somewhat curious that literature on applying grief therapy in treating the kinds of patients described in this book is essentially non-existent. The reasons for what seems an extraordinary gap in the literature on grief therapy does not lend itself to common sense. Loss is endemic among the population of patients who suffer from a chronic medical illness or disability. Coping with their grief in face of all they have lost is a daily struggle for patients who have experienced an amputation or who have become seriously compromised with respect to physical functioning. The literature describing the presence of grief in cancer patients is voluminous, and deserves a major review. But intervention strategies in helping these patients address their grief are scarcely reported. In an effort to overcome this shortcoming, we shall briefly review here the literature on grief therapy, such as it is, and then examine some possible ways to use grief therapy in treating patients whose losses are of a different order.

In Chapter 7 the treatment of an elderly person with multiple medical problems was discussed. This patient (Mrs Thomas) had to deal with the sudden death of her son and also the institutionalization of her husband because of his Alzheimer's disease. In the context of her life, the process of her grieving was described, as was the therapy used to help her cope with her losses. A brief review of the literature was provided. The main task in this chapter, however, is to explore, primarily through clinical illustrations, the journey that many of our type of patients undertake in coming to terms with their altered sense of self and redefined self-identity. At the core of the struggle for our patients is the everyday reality of the need to come to terms with their reduced physical capacity to perform the tasks required to maintain their routine, habitual, and self-esteem–sustaining roles. Loss of these roles is at the root of their despair. We looked at examples of the multitude of losses encountered by patients with chronic medical illness. Many of these losses occur suddenly. Others become manifest over many months and years. Losses resulting from disability or chronic medical illness may be permanent or transient. Some of these losses may be partially restored, such as regaining a higher level of physical functioning and ability to perform daily activities. Others are irreversible, as may be the case regarding employment or reduced financial circumstances. Helping patients not only to come to terms with their losses, but to maximize their residual abilities and in doing so find new directions and strengths is the purpose of grief therapy. Usually it is incorporated in the treatment plan along with many other interventions. Our experience leads us to recommend that the first task of a psychotherapist is to address the issues of identity that often confront patients who have become chronically ill or disabled.

GRIEF THERAPY

The task of finding a model of grief therapy to fit the requirements of people adjusting to a new set of realities in terms of their health problems and physical capabilities is a perilous one. The existing and widely used models for coping with grief focus on phases and tasks (Stroebe, Schut, and Stroebe, 1998). Their main purpose is 'decathexis of emotional energy from a loved one' (Neimeyer, 1999). These models are under considerable scrutiny, and they all are directly related to processing one's reactions upon the death of an intimate. Thus, they are of limited relevance to our primary focus. Furthermore, empirical support for these models is at best sketchy. Stroebe and colleagues (1998) described a model which they call 'loss-orientation and restoration-orientation.' Loss-orientation involves concentrating on or dealing with some particular aspects of the loss experience. Restoration-orientation addresses grieving the loss, but also the necessity to adjust to substantial changes that are secondary consequences of the loss. Bereavement following a death is used to illustrate their conceptualization. Nevertheless, this model can be applied to other kinds of losses where a redefinition of one's identity is called for. The strength of this model lies in its clear recognition that although grieving is an entirely normal and even necessary response to loss, a simultaneous requirement surfaces: the need to process the ensuing adjustment. We shall apply this model here in describing some of our own clinical endeavours.

LITERATURE REVIEW

Both the theoretical and the empirical literature on grief therapy will be considered here. Many authors are now claiming that grief therapy seems to be in the midst of a revolution. This is part and parcel of the current re-examination of the many precepts about grief, the roots of which may be traced back to Sigmund Freud. Neimeyer (1999) observed that some common elements of the new models are the following:

1. Scepticism regarding the predicability of the pathways leading from a state of disequilibrium to acceptance;
2. A shift away from letting go of the deceased (or any other particular loss as the case may be) to maintaining symbolic bonds with the lost 'object';
3. Attention to the meaning-making process in that mourning entails, as well as to the specific symptomatic and emotional consequences of the loss;
4. Attention to the altered identity of the bereaved;
5. Focus on the post-trauma (or post-loss) growth and integration of the lessons learned in connection with the loss;
6. Shifting the focus of loss from the bereaved individual to the entire family.

The effectiveness of grief therapy was examined by Allumbaugh and Hoyt (1999), in a meta-analysis of thirty-five outcome studies. They noted that the 'recently bereaved represent a large at-risk population, with higher overall death and suicide rates ... and with an increased incidence of depression, substance abuse, and certain medical disorders.' Before reviewing the findings, this paper also summarized the current types of grief therapy. Psychoanalytic approaches to grief are used, originally as proposed by Freud. These 'allow the bereaved to attribute the unfinished business of mourning to the therapist,' in what is called 'transference' (Allumbaugh and Hoyt, 1999), and work through guilt, which may be blocking the way to resolution. Implicit in this model is the notion of complicated or even abnormal, grief as the patient tries to resolve conflictual issues with the deceased.

Client-centred therapy is the other model that provides nurturance and support in addressing the patient's safety needs and overwhelming feelings of grief. Gestalt therapy serves a similar function through helping the patient come to terms with the dimensions of the loss. Cognitive therapy focuses on reversing the irrational thoughts and beliefs commonly observed in the bereaved by replacing them with rational beliefs. Behavioural therapy adopts a problem-solving approach in helping patients identify and define their problems, set goals, and find ways to realize these goals. With the exceptions of cognitive and behavioural therapies, all grief therapies are predicated on the time-honoured conceptualization of the grieving process, as articulated by neo-Freudians such as John Bowlby and Murray Parkes, and are rooted in the phase-tasks perspectives of grief therapy.

The key findings of Allumbaugh and Hoyt's (1999) the meta-analysis are complex, and it would be too simplistic to draw either a positive conclusion that grief therapy is generally effective or that it does not work. One critical observation was that individuals who seek treatment for bereavement issues benefit much more than 'small omnibus effect size produced by the meta analyses.' An explanation for this may be that individuals who seek treatment may have higher levels of distress than those who do not. Motivation may be higher in those seeking therapeutic help than 'those agreeing to treatment as a result of experimenter recruiting effort.' Another observation was that patients in both treatment and control groups experienced a time-lag before coming into treatment, and the healing process may have been well on its way before they entered therapy. Grief therapies with self-selected patients, which commenced within a few months of the loss experienced, was as effective or possibly more effective than was general psychotherapy. However, the precise lines of separation between grief therapy and psychotherapy were not altogether self-evident.

GRIEF THERAPY AND MEDICAL PROBLEMS

Unlike bereavement following a death, the loss of health may or may not be irretrievable. Even when loss involves amputation of a limb, rehabilitative treatment such as physical therapy and use of a prosthesis, may restore a good deal of the functioning. Altered body image, loss or change of employment, changes in family roles, and other, perhaps non-specific changes resulting from the loss of a limb constitute the core of grief therapy.

First, there are the actual losses and coming to terms with them. The loss is an insult to one's identity. It therefore becomes necessary to accept this new reality and 'reinvent' oneself. These are the goals of psychological interventions. Restoration of a sense of mastery or control over a specific or general loss due to chronic illness or disability would be seen as positive outcome. Many patients, in the face of serious and debilitating illness, continue to maintain a sense of control over their lives. One of our colleagues has multiple sclerosis. His illness advanced to the point where he could not sit for any length of time, and he found it hard to write in a supine position. Nevertheless, he wrote an entire book on his computer – standing up. Thompson and Kyle (2000) reported that chronically ill patients discover and adopt general strategies for keeping on top of their lives in face of serious difficulties. These general strategies involve acceptance, changing to reachable goals, finding and creating control, and using humour. Another strategy commonly used by chronic pain sufferers, who often can feel that their lives are totally controlled by pain, is engagement or focus. Our patients have frequently told us that in those moments when their minds are totally focused on something, perhaps while watching a favourite television show or good movie, they may become less aware of their pain or even oblivious to it. For those few minutes, they are controlling the pain instead of vice versa. Control is a central issue with a vast number of the patients seen in pain clinics.

In the only study of its kind, Whitley-Reed (1999) reported the results of grief therapy with a group of chronic pain sufferers with co-morbid depression. The approach used in treating this group employed an amalgam of several perspectives, but was in the main rooted in stage-tasks grief therapy. Treatment consisted of five weekly psychotherapy sessions. Sixty-one subjects were assigned to either a control or treatment group. Both groups received otherwise similar care, except that the treatment group also attended grief therapy. Overall, the results supported grief therapy as effective in reducing pain, the level of depression, the use of psychotropic drugs, and the number of visits to health care providers. Grief therapy enhanced patients' sense of well-being, motivated them to join rehabilitation programs, and improved their chances of returning to work. One major omission in this study was its failure to identify the types of losses experienced by the subjects. This was a serious drawback since it remains unclear what exactly these patients had lost and were grieving.

A small body of clinical literature has addressed the topic of grief therapy following amputation. All reports are anecdotal. They describe novel treatment approaches, for example, hospital-based grief therapy for a thirteen-year-year old boy after he had undergone an emergency amputation of his leg (Judd, 2001). Nau's report (1987) focused on the benefits of letter writing, for example, writing to one's lost (amputated) leg. Apparently, this method helped clients to confront their loss and grieve in a meaningful way. Buttenshaw (1993) described the entire rehabilitation process in detail, including psychological intervention for amputees. Grief therapy for cancer-related losses has been studied (Esplen et al., 2000; Fox and Rau, 2001; Hayashi, 1994; Swensen and Fuller, 1992). In these reports a variety of interventions are described: family-focused therapy, couples therapy, and in the case of an elderly patient, client-centred therapy using a life-review perspective.

Our brief review here suggests that physically ill patients benefit from grief therapy. The evidence is overwhelmingly clinical and anecdotal. However, grief related to death is a highly researched area and even there, as our review of the meta-analyses of that research showed, the findings are complex. Nevertheless, there was powerful evidence to support the contention that when patients seek grief therapy within a relatively short period after incurring their loss, the outcome is likely to be generally positive.

Grief associated with chronic physical illness, while bearing some resemblance to traumatic losses, has its own peculiarities. Losses often happen over some length of time. Many of the associated losses are predictable, giving patients time to reflect on their meaning and consequences. On occasions lost functions or roles are regained. But there also are irreversible losses. These variations often complicate the grieving process. In the case illustrations that follow, we hope to demonstrate two key issues that emerge again and again in the course of grief therapy with patients who have experienced a variety of physical problems and concomitant wide-ranging losses. The two issues are control and identity. Both of these issues have been addressed throughout this volume. However, it is worth reiterating that loss of control over one's functional abilities, and through that other losses, a redefinition of one's self becomes the essential goal of psychotherapeutic intervention. Grief therapy is designed to help patients develop some level of acceptance for their misfortune and to redirect their energy in discovering their capacity for change which ultimately will lead to a reintegration of self and a renewed identity.

LIVING WITH RHEUMATOID ARTHRITIS: MRS INNES

The case of Mrs Innes was described earlier in chapters 3 and 4. Her story encapsulates two central themes of grief therapy, namely, regaining a sense of control and redefining one's identity. To briefly recapitulate, Mrs Innes was diagnosed with juvenile rheumatoid arthritis while in her teens. When she was in her twenties she was referred to the pain clinic by her family physician for an investigation of her general mood. The referring physician was very concerned that coming to terms with her disease was posing a major challenge for Mrs Innes. The following is a summary of all the losses Mrs Innes encountered and the effects that these losses had on her identity.

Sudden Loss of Job

Mrs Innes had worked with animals at a veterinary hospital. To her mind, she had been dismissed unceremoniously by her employer for not being able to do her job. This was an enormous blow to her, and a great setback in her ongoing struggle in trying to minimize the effects of her rheumatoid arthritis on her life.

Loss of Physical Functions

Coping with her loss of physical functions was an ongoing struggle for Mrs Innes. She had no way of knowing how she might feel when she woke up in the morning. Some mornings her pain level was tolerable, and on others she had a hard time even getting out of bed. This uncertainty drove her to distraction and produced complex psychological responses. On days when she felt good, she was inclined to overdo it (for example, on one occasion she undertook to paint the outside of their home). The effect of this was severe pain and discomfort afterwards that lasted for several days. She also engaged in what may be described as counterphobic behaviour, always testing her strength and usually suffering as a consequence.

Loss of Social Roles

Mrs Innes did not have a large circle of friends. With the passage of time, she more or less withdrew from all her outside activities and became very unsure about all her relationships with people. She basically retreated into her domestic world which was periodically intruded upon by her very caring parents.

Compromised Spousal Role

Mrs Innes's pain interfered with many of her domestic as well as conjugal roles and functions. She was married to a very caring and understanding man who made no demands on her. On the contrary, her husband quietly assumed most of the responsibilities for running the household, ensuring that his wife did not have to exert herself unnecessarily. But this had two sides for Mrs Innes. Certainly, she was deeply appreciative of her husband's consideration. However, she felt ridden with guilt for not being able to pull what she thought was her weight. This guilt was compounded by her awareness that she and her husband had greatly reduced their sexual activities with each other, as she found sexual intercourse caused her much discomfort and pain. As a partner, she felt inadequate and at times entirely useless.

All of these losses amounted to loss of her dream of working with animals, her once-happy marriage, her sense of control over her life. She found herself feeling increasingly at the mercy of her disease and pain. When her disease was quiet, however, she would become unduly optimistic. As the disease became active again, there would be a corresponding loss of hope. When she arrived at our pain clinic, she was in a state of deep despair.

Considered together, all these losses had profoundly shaken her sense of who and what she was. Mrs Innes was young, but she did not have the physical strength of a person of her age. She was a woman, and a wife, and in both respects felt seriously compromised. She had been an active member of the workforce, but this was no longer held true. When Mrs Innes was first seen, her sense of self and identity was in a state of total flux, causing her great anguish.

The Therapeutic Process

Mrs Innes was in psychotherapy for a year and a half. The therapeutic process in which she was engaged will be analysed in terms of a strategy oriented towards loss-restoration. Loss-orientation is a focus on the losses experienced. In Mrs Innes's case, there were many. For the first several initial sessions, Mrs Innes said very little and mostly wept quietly. She never missed a session, and she was never late. Nevertheless, these early sessions were characterized by much silence. It seemed that Mrs Innes, until coming to the clinic, had not allowed herself to show any external signs of grief, and when she finally did, all her sadness just poured right out of her.

For the next several months, she had two distinct sources of preoccupation. First was what amounted to almost an obsession with her blood test taken each month which revealed her disease activity. Second was the virtually overwhelming humiliation she experienced at being fired from her job. Gradually, Mrs Innes's range of focus expanded to include the whole gamut of the losses that had deprived her of any and all sense of the meaning or purpose of her life. During this entire phase, Mrs Innes remained very negative and sad. This is where her self-esteem was lowest.

The restoration phase began almost imperceptibly for Mrs Innes. One of the very early signs of it was her ability on 'good' days to engage in activities to a measured degree, rather than overdoing it and then suffering afterwards. This was an indication of an effort on her part to begin to acknowledge her disease and recognize the limits it imposed on her and her lifestyle. At this time, Mrs Innes decided to inform herself about rheumatoid arthritis. This was another positive sign. Mrs Innes was beginning to regain some sense of control over her situation.

Mr Innes had his own business, and Mrs Innes now began to take more than a passing interest in it. Her weeping during therapy virtually ceased. Sometimes she would even tell the therapist stories showing her deep love of horses and of her experiences in working with animals. One day, quite unexpectedly, Mrs Innes announced to the therapist that, unbeknown to him, she had been volunteering at a local childcare facility for a couple of hours a day for the past two weeks and that she was very much enjoying her interaction with the children there.

These were all early signs of reintegration, which came about through her search for meaningful new activities. The long process of redefining her identity had started. During the last phase of her therapy, Mrs Innes began taking an active role in her husband's business. She took over handling all his appointments and acting as the office manager. She decided to upgrade her computer skills so that she could handle his accounts. By the termination point of her therapy, Mrs Innes had completed the computer course and was actively involved in many aspects of the business.

Mrs Innes achieved two essential goals during her therapy. First, she came to terms with having to live with a chronic and potentially progressive illness. Second, she found meaningful alternative activities and thus was able to begin the process of creating a somewhat revised identity for herself. Her self-esteem was restored to a very significant degree. She was very fortunate in her partner, not only for his support and love for her, but because he had a business in which she could imagine a role. This provided the incentive and opportunity that Mrs Innes needed to begin her recovery process. Mrs Innes, in all probability, will continue to struggle with her disease and all its changes and their ramifications for the rest of her life. And she will probably do so successfully, having already shown considerable resilience in confronting her disease and find new meaning in her life. At the point of discharge, Mrs Innes was advised to contact the clinic should she ever felt the need to do so. She has not made contact since. At the time of this writing, that was four years ago.

PAIN AND TRAUMATIC LOSS: MRS DAVIES

Mrs Davies (see Chapter 2) was born into a middle-class family, the elder of the two siblings. Her father was a bank manager and her mother a homemaker. Her developmental milestones all followed a normal progression, and she recalled her childhood as 'not particularly unhappy.' However, Mrs Davies revealed that her father was a very cold, distant, and authoritarian individual who tended to be a heavy-handed disciplinarian. He never physically abused his two daughters, but found novel ways of punishing them and also had extremely high expectations of them. It was almost impossible for Mrs Davies and her sister to live up to these expectations, and they constantly felt they were letting their father down. In contrast, their mother was a warm and gentle person, who in her quiet way exerted some influence on her husband and attempted to curb his unusual and unrealistic demands on the children. Mrs Davies had been very close to her mother throughout her childhood years and maintained that closeness until her mother died. According to Mrs Davies, it was her mother who enabled her to grow up in a reasonably normal way and maintain her sanity.

Although Mrs Davies's growing-up years were strained, she did not suffer from any particular problem with pain. The first sign of her headaches appeared when she was fourteen years old, and it coincided with the onset of menses. Initially, the headaches were not particularly severe. They lasted a short time and usually cleared up spontaneously. But the headaches worsened, and by the time Mrs Davies was twenty, she was having fairly regular and severe headaches. She was living alone and working, and the headaches had already begun to interfere with her social activities, although not with her work. She consulted her own physician and a number of specialists, but the pain did not abate. Despite her problems, Mrs Davies viewed herself as a reasonably healthy young woman and tried to live as normal a life as circumstances would allow.

At the age of twenty-four, Mrs Davies married a man she had known for two years. From the very outset the marriage ran into difficulties because of her headaches. In the main the headaches interfered quite seriously with the couple's social life. In addition, there were times when Mrs Davies was incapacitated by her head pain, and her husband had to assume major responsibilities for looking after the household and their two young children, in addition to holding down a demanding job. This created a lot of tension between the two over the years, but they never sought any professional assistance. The only help obtained was for the headaches, but for all practical purposes Mrs Davies did not benefit from medical treatment.

Throughout her married life Mrs Davies felt that her husband was 'cheated' because of her poor health. The marriage was further characterized by dissension and disagreement concerning the raising of the children. Mr Davies was a tolerant and lenient, if not permissive, person who had a disregard for any kind of discipline. His views were in direct conflict with Mrs Davies's, as she was inclined to be strict. To complicate the situation further, Mr Davies worked different shifts. Mrs Davies held his irregular work hours against her husband throughout their life together, but never did any thing about it, such as talking to him about it.

The couple had their share of problems with their children. The older of the two, a daughter, did not present any serious difficulties until her late teens. However, according to Mrs Davies, their son was 'spoiled' by his father, had serious problems at school, and had failed many subjects. He was also involved in serious antisocial activities, such as minor theft and driving without a licence.

When Mrs Davies was fifty-four years old, her husband died suddenly and unexpectedly. He returned home from work, rang the doorbell, and then had a massive heart attack and died on the spot. Following his death. Mrs Davies's headaches became extremely severe. This development coincided with increased antisocial activity on the part of her son, who was apprehended for drunken driving and for not having a licence. At this point, the son decided to move out of the house and to start living with an older woman of whom Mrs Davies did not approve. In the meantime, her daughter had become restless, hard to reach, and aimless. All this became unbearable for Mrs Davies, who while in these circumstances was referred to a pain clinic with extremely severe and unabating headaches.

Losses

It was unclear at the point of Mrs Davies's initial visit to our clinic what some of her problems were. Her letter of referral was only about her increasingly severe headaches. When the fact of the death of her husband some two years previous came to light, it was at first unclear whether there were unresolved issues surrounding his untimely death.

It was some time before the full impact of her husband's death on Mrs Davies began to be appreciated. She had profoundly conflicting views about her marriage. Bit by bit, her husband had more or less taken over every aspect of their family life. This had happened over many years and was, in part, as a result of her headaches. Mrs Davies did appreciate his help, but at the same time resented the fact that the family hardly needed her. This conflict manifested mainly as unresolved anger towards her dead husband. The other prominent emotion was one of feeling abandoned. She felt that her husband had abandoned her by dying.

Another critical factor that came to light was that Mrs Davies's health and family situation had worsened since the death of her husband. Her family was coming apart at the seams, and Mrs Davies was responding to this situation with more severe and more frequent headaches. The losses for Mrs Davies were monumental. She lost her husband, her health, the well-being of her children, and was witnessing the virtual dissolution of her family. In sum, she lost many of her roles, except the role of being chronically sick, which instead became even more pronounced. In her mind, Mrs Davies had not only failed to fill the vacuum left by her husband's death, but her situation had worsened to the point of utter hopelessness. Other than her anger in reaction to her husband's sudden death, she showed very few overt signs of grief. Nevertheless, it was undeniable that since her husband's death, she had sunk deeper and deeper into the chronic sick role.

Goals of Therapy

The therapeutic process had two clear goals. The first was to enable Mrs Davies to come to terms with her losses. The second was to begin the process of restoration. During the first few months of therapy much of the information about Mrs Davies's life and circumstances was obtained. It was also during this phase that she began to express regrets about having turned so many of her responsibilities over to her husband over the years. She felt that she was a failure as a mother and that she had not been much of a wife. Mrs Davies dwelled for a long time on these failures. She began to appreciate that the combination of having chronic headaches and a very caring and responsible husband had unwittingly, and through no one's fault eroded some of her key roles. One role, that of a partner and spouse, was irretrievably lost, but others could still be salvaged.

Early in her treatment at our clinic, Mrs Davies also participated in a cognitive-behavioural group therapy program. She began to develop a sense of control not only over her headaches, but also over her life in general. A major focus of her therapy was to enable Mrs Davies to work through her anger and mixture of emotions in relation to her late husband. She came to accept that he had been a good man and that she had been overly reliant on him, which at the end had cost her much. Perhaps, however, Mr Davies had not been solely responsible for that state of affairs.

The question of restoration of roles for Mrs Davies was complicated. Her parental role was seriously compromised. Both her children were already young adults. It became a challenge for her to determine whether any kind of relationship could be restored. She had more success with her daughter. Over time, Mrs Davies managed to motivate her daughter to return to school. This she did by gradually taking an interest in her daughter's affairs, creating an environment where the daughter felt free to talk about her father and what losing him meant to her. In therapy, Mrs Davies recalled her own close relationship with her mother, and made it her goal to develop such a relationship with her daughter.

The problem with Mrs Davies's son was more serious. He came and went as he pleased. He did not seem to have any boundaries. Mrs Davies gained sufficient confidence to convey to him that if he was to live under her roof, she expected him to abide by her rules. This process of connecting with her son was prolonged and not entirely successful.

For the first time in her life, except for the brief period before her marriage, Mrs Davies began to take charge of her family's finances. Her husband had left her well provided for. Financial management was a major challenge for a woman who had never even paid a bill or had any concern with money matters. Taking over this role significantly increased her self-confidence. She began to form close friendships with two women from her group therapy program. In addition, she reconnected with her sister, with whom her relationship had, at best, been tenuous over the years.

Mrs Davies remained in therapy for about two years. By the end of that time, she had regained much of the confidence and self-reassurance that she had once possessed as a young woman. She thought it was ironic that it took her husband's death for her to find herself.

TOO MUCH TO BEAR: MS. PETERS

Ms. Peters (see Chapter 6) was in her teens at the time of her referral to our pain clinic. She complained of persistent lower abdominal pain that she had been experiencing following hysterectomy and vaginoplasty. At the time of her referral she was struggling with identity issues. She had lost her ability to have children, and this at such a critical stage in her development. Ms. Peters showed herself as filled with anxiety mixed with feelings of loss over her compromised self-image and emerging womanhood. She was overwhelmed by a sense of not belonging. She shied away from her peer group and expressed very confusing and contradicting wishes. Ms. Peters wanted to belong and feel part of her peer group. At the same time, she regarded her peers as lacking compassion and understanding. She knew suffering at first-hand, having watched her young friends in hospital die. What could she possibly have in common with her school mates who were preoccupied with clothes and boyfriends?

Ms. Peters's feelings of loss were mixed with feelings of guilt. She was convinced, as was her family, that her 'loss of womanhood' was some kind of divine retribution. This was very much a belief held by both her parents. When Ms. Peters first came for therapy her entire preoccupation was 'Why did it have to happen to me?'

Ms. Peters, at the time of this writing, has been in therapy for over a year. During this period she had shown remarkable resiliency both in coping with her ongoing pain problem and with conflicts centring on her identity. In the very early stages of therapy, her parents were seen by the therapist to address their issues and concern and to gauge the level of support Ms. Peters had from them. The parents were indeed extraordinarily supportive of their daughter. It became evident that the mother, in particular, was Ms. Peters's main source of support. They had a very trusting and close relationship. The question of their belief that Ms. Peters's loss of reproductive organs somehow amounted to divine retribution was discussed. The parents were asked to consider the consequences for their daughter not having had the surgeries, and the real possibility that Ms. Peters's prognosis would have been seriously compromised. The parents agreed that they had been so preoccupied with the harsh reality of their daughter never becoming a mother that they had not given any thought to any of the other possible outcomes of their daughter's health problems. They agreed that Ms. Peters was much better off for having had the surgeries, and that they had to convey with conviction that message to their daughter. Over time Ms. Peters's conviction that she was being punished lost its hold on her considerably.

Treatment

In therapy, Ms. Peters gradually gave up her preoccupation with the loss of her uterus. She began to show concerns that were more congruent with those of a teenager. She worried about her looks, about her clothes, and about her friends. She insisted that she was too young to have a boyfriend, but nevertheless she got along quite well with boys. There was a significant shift in her attitude towards her peers. She became less judgmental of them. Ms. Peters had a small group of close friends and generally got along with most young people. She was no longer bothered about her peers. In short, she no longer felt like much of an outsider. It was this sense that she was not all that different from her peers, after all, which is so very important for an adolescent, that may be viewed as the turning point in Ms. Peter's therapy. Her grades improved, and she began to give serious thought to pursuing a medical career. On a day-to-day basis, there was little evidence of any anxiety or preoccupation with her health and body image, other than her appearance. At the time of this writing, Ms. Peters remains in therapy, and is seen once every two weeks. She continues to make excellent progress.

Analysis

Several aspects of this case are noteworthy. First, there is the nature of her loss. The loss of her reproductive capacity was irretrievable. Second, her faith contributed significantly to her belief in divine retribution, and this was initially reinforced by her parents. Third was the relevance of her developmental stage, early to mid-adolescence, when she had to undergo the surgeries – and their impact on her self-image. Fourth, the surgeries had social consequences for her and affected her peer relationships and in some ways slowed her developmental progression. Ms. Peters looked and behaved much more like an eleven-year-old than a fourteen-year-old when she was first seen.

Neither the phase-task based perspective nor the loss-restoration paradigm was altogether applicable in treating Ms. Peters. For this patient, the major task was and remains to grow into an adult without a permanent sense of loss and without feeling any less of a person or a woman because of her inability to conceive a child. This is not just a matter of restoring her lost roles, if anticipated rather than experienced roles, or of helping her to go through well-defined phases of grieving to arrive at some resolution. Rather, this young woman has embarked on a journey that has no well-defined end-points. Who can predict whether she will not have a renewed sense of grief over the loss of her ability to bear children when she becomes old enough to have a family? One can only hope that her current therapy will prepare her, to a degree, for such contingencies and enable her to cope with them with some degree of acceptance and resiliency.

CONCLUSION

A major challenge that many patients with chronic medical illness or disability face is their confusion in regard to the nature and the extent of their losses. This is because many of their losses may not be temporary or at least partially recoverable. Also, often their losses do not descend upon them all at once, but incrementally over time, as the disease worsens or for other reasons they become unable to maintain their previous levels of functioning and previous roles. This process is unpredictable, which, in turn, poses special problems in therapy. In the face of an unpredictable illness, it is impossible to know what losses may be incurred and when in the future. For these reasons, much of the therapeutic effort has to be focused on recognizing these very facts, and at the same time on optimizing the abilities and resources and roles that are available to the patient. The therapy literature is silent on the problem of coming to terms with the loss ensuing from chronic illness, and the conventional literature on bereavement is of little relevance.

The three cases presented in this chapter highlight the problems of determining the end point of therapy. Regaining some of her valued roles was important for Mrs Innes, and her medical condition was such that any dramatic and sudden deterioration was not very likely. The situations were more complicated with the two other patients.

Mrs Innes had rheumatoid arthritis, a disease with an unpredictable course. The ultimate consequences of Ms. Peters's loss, namely, the ability to have children, were as yet far into the future for her. However, both these patients were also concerned with immediate issues. Traditional grief therapy, which focuses on coming to terms with the death of a loved one, was not altogether applicable. The phase-task approach or the loss-restoration approach to working through grief were relevant.

Coming to terms with a disease with unknown course for Mrs Innes and a loss that could have its greatest impact only later in her life for fourteen-year-old Ms. Peters were losses not amenable to conclusive resolution. The phases that are normally associated with grieving could not be applied in the aftermath of these losses because there were no well-defined end points to their grief experiences. Furthermore, there could very well remain for them more losses associated with the illness or the surgeries, respectively, to cope with in the future. At this time in their lives the tasks involved regaining equilibrium and a redefined positive identity in face of their experiences of loss – loss of work and diminished physical functioning for one patient, and profound feelings of being different from her peers, who had not lost their reproductive organs, for the other.

Identity issues, in many ways, defined the struggle of both women. Coming to terms with their altered sense of self led to a reasonable outcome of therapy in both cases. Mrs Innes found a new career, and young Ms. Peters rediscovered her adolescence with all its ecstasies and agonies. What the future holds for these two patients is unknown. There are no longitudinal outcome studies to give us any guidance. There is often a more or less clear starting point to this grieving process, but the end point is unpredictable, both as to its nature and timing. Indeed, our reports of success must be viewed with caution as they are purely anecdotal. There is a clear need for experimentation and research to discover what may be construed as common elements shared by chronically ill patients. There may be none. Perhaps, an argument can be made that identity issues are commonly found in the chronically ill population. Some loss of functioning is also common. Although touched on here, and in earlier chapters, a major omission in this chapter is a thorough analysis of the role of the family of our patients in their therapy. In any event, the need for specialized grief therapy for the population of patients with a chronic medical illness or disability can hardly be exaggerated.

The grief literature is astonishingly lacking with regard to some of the issues raised in this book. There is a great need for explicit articulation of grief therapy as it applies to the particular and very complex ongoing process of grieving for the losses experienced by those of us who are chronically ill.

10

Epilogue

The paramount aim in writing this book has been to find some ways in which to convey the sheer variability and complexity that any general discussion of chronic medical illness presents. Chronic illness encompasses a wide and complex array of disorders and an equally complex range of patient responses to them. Many patients with debilitating diseases continue to function at a high level, while at the other end are patients with persistent pain of unknown of origin who become virtually completely disabled. They all experience losses ensuing from their chronic health condition; they all react to their losses in one way or another. A further complication is that, as we have seen with several patients described in this book, some losses are regained and some are not. Some patients are able to redefine themselves and, ultimately, find acceptance of their new selves; others are not.

Undeniably, chronic illness can lead to a multitude of losses. Insult to the person's identity as a result of chronic diseases may be a common occurrence. The degree and depth of insult vary considerably among such patients, but it should be assumed that chronic illness is going to present a challenge to the patient's sense of self. Awareness of this fundamental fact offers an opportunity to begin the process of assessing the losses that each particular patient experiences – not merely by identifying and then adding up the tangible losses, but by identifying the consequences of the illness on the patient's sense of self.

Many patients, in the face of the enormous upheaval in their lives brought on by their illness, remain relatively calm and are able to achieve, better than resignation, acceptance. Their sense of loss does not overwhelm them. Their identity, their sense of who and what they are, basically remain intact. This reaction was observed in the study of elderly people with pain problems living in the community. These people took their pain in stride, modified their activities accordingly, perhaps, and generally maintained very good mental health and continued to be involved with the outside world. The predominant attitude, it seemed, was that pain is a common problem in the elderly, and that one could not simply become a recluse because of pain. Age was undoubtedly a factor. Nevertheless, these people were secure in their identity, and they seemed to take the view that to live with one or many conditions causing pain was hardly a reason to retreat from life.

Losses are many, as well as endemic among people with chronic illness. Some are permanent, others restorable. Still others require life course adjustments, such as retraining for a new type of job. The quality of these losses makes them similar to and also different from the loss related to the death of a loved one. This qualitative distinction poses a challenge to the notion of any general theory of loss and grief. Response to loss, whether it be as a result of a death, the sudden loss of employment, the loss of a limb to amputation, or the loss of one's family and social roles, is more than likely to be sadness and grief. All losses entail some form of grieving. Whatever the loss and whatever the reaction to it, there exists the potential possibility that the grieving process may go awry.

The loss and grief literature is so deeply attached to the grief that follows a death that much of it does not directly apply to the topic at hand. It would be difficult and not particularly appropriate to use the notion of stages of grief in addressing the losses experienced by many of our patients. For many patients with a chronic illness, loss of their job is by far the most devastating from among their losses, and its consequences are far reaching. Job loss may be permanent, but not necessarily and not always. There are too many permutations and computations to make job loss, even when resulting from chronic and debilitating illness, comparable to the death of a loved one. Weiss (1998) pointed out that there are many kinds of loss, with varied responses and outcomes. He questions the utility of applying the time-honoured phase-task approach to resolving grief across the board. Weiss proposed three categories of losses: (1) loss through death of critically important relationships, for example, the death of a spouse; (2) losses that challenge self-esteem and diminish self-worth, for example, job loss; and (3) losses through victimization through criminal acts such as robbery, battery, or rape, which can result in loss of self-respect and social humiliation. This view contradicts much of our contemporary understanding of grief, where one loss is considered to need the same kind of grief process as another, where grief in response to the loss of a limb is taken to be analogous to the loss of a spouse – if different in magnitude.

Weiss's classification has its problems. Nevertheless, it provides a conceptual starting point for a theoretical discourse on grief and chronic illness. Loss of any kind can engender depression and even suicide. Most people, however, do find ways of coming to terms with the death of someone they love dearly, and most chronically ill patients manage to live with their losses somehow. I am currently working with a woman who with is slowly losing her sight. So far it has been a gradual process. She was devastated when she first learned that she would go blind. Soon after she began attending a group therapy program at her local centre for the blind. The hardest part of this, she says, is for her to watch people she has come to know lose their sight. Yet at the same time she is constantly reassured by their capacity to get on with their lives, and even learn to accept their blindness – an outcome for our patient that she, too, hopes to achieve when the time comes.

One issue that remains relatively untouched and certainly is underresearched is the phenomenon of abnormal grief in relation to people who are chronically ill. What markers determine that someone has failed utterly to accept the loss (or losses) emanating from a chronic disorder? The normal clinical signs associated with abnormal or pathological grief all concern grief following death. They include, for example, the grievers' failure to believe that the person whose absence they are grieving really is dead, or they remain stuck in immobilizing grief long after the death, or they fail to return to some modicum of normal day-to-day living after the passage of some reasonable length of time. Many of these behaviours are simply not applicable as markers of grief gone awry in the experience and behaviour of people coming to terms with their own chronic illness. Even the loss of a limb, while traumatic, may not be a total loss; prosthetics often restore significant functions. The loss of some valued role, such as one's sexual role through loss of libido or even impotence because of diabetics does not follow a parallel course among individuals, nor a course parallel to the grieving process normally associated with bereavement. There seem to be a variety of pathways that may be taken by individuals who are chronically ill in coming to terms with their losses and moving beyond them.

Clinically observable behavioural markers do exist that suggest a patient is coming to terms with the loss she or he has experienced and is even moving on. This was evident in a number of the cases described in this book. What is more difficult to determine is the timeline that as practitioners we so firmly, and perhaps somewhat erroneously, seem to want to link to the grieving process. The loss and crisis literature emphasizes the significance of time, not so much in overcoming the loss, but as a desire on the part of both the bereaved and the therapist as a marker signifying when precisely it would be appropriate to resume normal living. The very idea of normal living for many chronically ill patients is a contradiction in terms, an impossibility, given the particular illness. No one expects a recently paralysed individual to return to any semblance of normalcy in six or eight weeks. Nevertheless, we, as yet, do not have any firm or even not so firm guidelines to assess healthy as opposed to unhealthy adaptations that a person may be making to the loss of all feeling below the waist. The struggle in making such adaptations is ongoing and may last from many months to many years.

Consequently, there is a tendency to equate grief with depression. Even a decade ago this debate was very evident in the chronic pain literature. The inclination was to overdiagnose depression in this population. Rather then taking into account their responses to the many losses they had endured and view their attitude as one of grieving, the tendency and indeed the practice was to diagnose them with a psychiatric disorder.

The dilemma of assessing success in rehabilitation is well illustrated by the debate surrounding what constitutes a positive treatment outcome for patients with chronic low-back pain. Return to work is viewed as the most desirable goal by practitioners in most pain management clinics. For many patients, however, return to work may be a goal that is unattainable. Failure to meet this objective becomes a source of great sorrow and shame for these patients. Society's definition of a successful outcome may be at variance with an individual's capacity, usually at a great cost to the individual. This scenario illustrates that (1) a loss such as job-loss may be viewed as not permanent when indeed it is; (2) recovery from a medical condition, in this instance chronic pain, is directly related to the restoration of a valued role, namely, employment; and (3) failure to achieve the goal of returning to gainful employment is considered to be the fault of the patients. For many of these patients, failure means revictimization, and the ensuing depression and hopelessness is what we see in them. It is a mistake to think that one treatment fits all and that those who fail to benefit are simply treatment failures. There is no parallel to this process in the bereavement literature. If this line of logic is followed then the bereaved are to be held responsible for being affected by their loss, and if they fail to attain some predetermined goal of treatment, they are to be held responsible for non-compliance, with their treatment regimen, and so on.

For many chronically ill and disabled individuals, treatment and recovery are measured in terms of restoration of lost roles, and not much attention is paid to the psychological impact of their losses, or on even rarer instances, does an adequate assessment seem to be made of the residual abilities of the patient. This may be termed the 'functional approach' to loss: Restore as much as you can of what has been lost, and your patient is well on the way to recovery.

The concept of 'chronic sick role' may be some value in this discussion. The proposition being made here is that although chronic illness is likely to compromise many customary roles and functions, the goal of treatment is to maximize the patient's residual abilities. Loss-orientation and restoration-orientation as an approach to the treatment of grief in this population may have its roots in the chronic sick role. First, identify the nature and extent of losses experienced and then determine which roles and functions can be restored or acquired. This perspective provides a cursory blueprint for an intervention strategy with patients who have a chronic illness or disability.

Chronic illness in all its manifestations can be the cause of enormous losses and grief. In this book, we have made an attempt to explore the scope of grief and chronic illness and begin the process of sorting out important differences and similarities between different kinds of losses. We have taken very preliminary and tentative steps to show the benefits of grief therapy that is not so much rooted in psychodynamic theory, but far more in a combination of the psychology of the individual under discussion and that individual's social environment.

The remaining question is perhaps the most important one. How sensitive are we, as healthcare professionals, in recognizing loss and grief in our chronically ill patients? Often, we take their sorrow and depression as normal and obvious responses. Only rarely, it seems, do we concern ourselves with the serious challenge that a chronic illness or disability presents to such a patient's very identity and that this assault on the patient's identity may require our attention and even therapeutic interventions.

References

Abraido-Lanza, A.-F. (1997). Latinas with arthritis: Effects of illness, role identity, and competence on psychological well-being. *American Journal of Community Psychology*, 25: 601–27.

Adams, S., Pill, R., and Jones, A. (1997). Medication, chronic illness and identity: The perspective of people with asthma. *Social Science and Medicine*, 45: 189–201.

Akechi,T., Okamura, H., Yamawani, S., and Uchitomi. Y. (2001). Why do some cancer patients with depression desire an early death and others do not? *Psychosomatics*, 42: 141–5.

Alarcon, N. (1994). The role of healthcare professionals in increasing access to primary health care. *Family and Community Health*, 17: 15–21.

Allanbaugh, D., and Hoyt, W. (1999). Effectiveness of grief therapy: A meta analysis. *Journal of Counseling Psychology*, 46: 370–80.

Allebeck, P., and Bolund, C. (1991). Suicide and suicide attempts in cancer patients. *Psychological Medicine*, 21: 979–84.

Allumbaugh, D., and Hoyt, W. (1999). Effectiveness of grief therapy: A meta-analysis. *Journal of Counselling Psychology*, 46: 370–80.

Almgren, G., Guest, A., Immerwahr, G., and Spittal, M. (1998). Joblessness, family disruption, and violent death in Chicago, 1970–1990. *Social-Forces*, 76: 1465–93.

Alonzo, A. (2000). The experience of chronic illness and post-traumatic stress disorder: The consequences of cumulative adversity. *Social Science and Medicine*, 50: 1475–84.

Amir, M., Neumann, L., Bor, O., Shir, Y., Rubinow, A., and Buskila, D. (2000). Coping styles, anger, social support, and suicide risk of women with fibromyalgia syndrome. *Journal of Musculoskeletal Pain*, 8: 7–20.

Ammerman, R., and Hersen, M. (1992). Current issues in the assessment of family violence. In R. Ammerman and M. Hersen (Eds.). *Assessment of family violence: A clinical and legal sourcebook*. New York: Wiley.

Ananth, J. (1983). Hysterectomy and sexual counselling. *Psychiatric Journal of the University of Ottawa*, 8: 213–17.

Andelman, F. (2001). Analysis of quality of life among adolescents with epilepsy. *International Journal of Adolescent Medicine and Health*, 112 (Suppl.): S17–S24.

Anderson, B., and Le Grand, J. (1991). Body image for women: Conceptualization, assessment, and a test of its importance to sexual dysfunction and medical illness. *Journal of Sex Research*, 28: 457–78.

Anderson, H., Ejlertsson, G., Leden, I., and Rosenberg, C. (1996). Chronic pain in a geographically defined population: Studies of differences in age, gender, social class, and pain localization. *Clinical Journal of Pain*, 9: 174–82.

Archer, J., and Rhodes, V. (1993). The grief process and job loss: A cross-sectional study. *British Journal of Psychology*, 84: 395–410.

Arluke, A. (1988). The sick-role concept. In D. Gochman (Ed.), *Health behavior: Emerging research perspectives*. New York: Plenum.

Averill, P., Novy, D., Nelson, D., and Berry, L. (1996). Correlates of depression in chronic pain patients: A comprehensive examination. *Pain*, 65: 93–100.

Banks, S., and Kearns, R. (1996). Explaining high rates of depression in chronic pain: A diathesis-stress framework. *Psychological Bulletin*, 119: 95–110.

Barbato, A., and Irwin, H. (1992). Major therapeutic systems and the bereaved client. *Australian Psychology*, 27: 22–7.

Barling, J. (1990). *Employment, stress and family functioning*. New York: Wiley.

Barlow, J., Cullen, L., Foster, N., Harmson, K., and Wade, M. (1999). Does arthritis influence perceived ability to fulfil a parenting role? Perceptions of mothers, fathers and grandmothers. *Patient Education and Counselling*, 37: 141–51.

Barron, W. (1997). Pain-prone theory: Interrelationships between childhood abuse history and chronic pain in adults. *Dissertation Abstracts International: Section B – Sciences and Engineering*, 57 (12B): 7715.

Bartos, M., and McDonald, K. (2000). HIV as identity, experience or career. *AIDS Care*, 3: 299–306.

Bedard, M., Raney, D., Molloy, D., Lever, J., Pedlar, D., and Dubois, S. (2001). The experience of primary and secondary caregivers caring for the same adult with Alzheimer's disease. *Journal of Mental Health and Aging*, 2: 287–96.

Bengesser, G. (1998). Pain, suicide, and its prevention. *Nordic Journal of Psychiatry*, 52: 183–4.

Bennett, K. (1997). Widowhood in elderly women: The medium and long-term effects on mental and physical health. *Mortality*, 2: 137–48.

Bernhard, L. (1985). Black woman's concerns about sexuality and hysterectomy. *Sage: A Scholarly Journal on Black women*, 2: 25–7.

Bhatia, M., Kaur, N., Bohra, N., and Goyal, U. (1990). Psychiatric reactions in hysterectomy. *Indian Journal of Psychiatry*, 32: 52–6.

Bhojak, M., Nathawat, S., and Swami, D. (1989). Psychological consequences following lower limb amputation. *Indian Journal of Clinical Psychology*, 1: 102–4.

Blake, D., Maisiak, R., Brown, S., and Koplan, A. (1986). Acceptance by arthritis patients of clinical inquiry into their sexual adjustment. *Psychosomatics*, 27: 576–9.

Bleich, C., and Witte, E. (1992). Changes in the couple relationship during unemployment of the male partner. *Kölner-Zeitschrift für Soziologie*, 44: 731–46.

Bonnanno, G., Keltner, D., Holen, A., and Horowitz, M. (1995). When avoiding unpleasant emotions might not be such a bad thing: Verbal automic response dissociation and midlife conjugal bereavement. *Journal of Personality and Social Psychology*, 5: 975–89.

Bouras, N., Vanger, P., and Bridges, P. (1986). Marital problems in chronically depressed and physically ill patients and their spouses. *Comprehensive Psychiatry*, 27: 127–30.

Bowlby, J. (1981). *Attachment and loss*, Vol. 3: *Loss, sadness, and depression*. Harmondsworth: Penguin.

Brauhn, N.E.H. (1999). Phenomenology of having HIV/AIDS at a time when medical advances are improving prognosis. *Dissertation Abstracts International: Section A – Humanities and Social Science*, 60(2A): 0346.

Bromberger, J., and Matthews, K. (1994). Employment status and depressive symptoms in middle-aged women: A longitudinal investigation. *American Journal of Public Health*, 84: 202–6.

Bruce, M. (1999). The association between depression and disability. *American Journal of Geriatric Psychiatry*, 7: 8–11.

Buttenshaw, P. (1993). Rehabilitation of the elderly lower limb amputee. *Reviews in Clinical Gerontology*, 3: 69–84.

Cacioppo, J., Poehlmann, K., Kiecolt-Glaser, J., et al. (1998). Cellular immune responses to acute stress in female caregivers of dementia patients and matched controls. *Health Psychology*, 17: 182–9.

Carnelley, K., Wortman, C., and Kessler. R. (1999). The impact of widowhood on depression: Findings from a prospective survey. *Psychological Medicine*, 29: 1111–23.

Carr, D., House, J., Kessler, R., Nesse, R., Sonnega, J., and Wortman, C. (2000). Marital quality and psychological adjustment to widowhood among older adults: A longitudinal analysis. *Journals of Gerontology: Series B – Psychological Sciences and Social Sciences*, 55B: S197–S207.

Charmaz, K. (1999). From the 'sick role' to stories of self: Understanding the self in illness. In R. Contrade, and R. Ashmore (Eds.), *Self, social identity and physical health* (pp. 209–39). New York: Oxford University Press.

Christoffersen, M. (1994). A follow-up study of long term effects of unemployment on children: Loss of self-esteem and self-destructive behavior among adolescents. *Childhood: A Global Journal of Child Research*, 2: 212–20.

– (2000). Growing up with unemployment: A study of parental unemployment and children's risk of abuse and neglect based on national longitudinal 1973 birth cohorts in Denmark. *Childhood: A Global Journal of Child Research*, 7: 421–38.

Ciaramella, A., and Poli, P. (2001). Assessment of depression among cancer patients: The role of pain, cancer type and treatment. *Psycho-Oncology*, 10: 156–65.

Clark, W. (1996). The stress of job loss upon both partners in a marital relationship. *Dissertation Abstracts International: Section B – Sciences and Engineering*, 57(3B): 2217.

Claussen, B., Bjorndal, A., and Hjort, P. (1993). Health and reemployment in a two-year follow-up of long term unemployment. *Journal of Epidemiology and Community Health*, 47: 14–18.

Clayton, P. (1974). Mortality and morbidity in the first year of widowhood. *Archives of General Psychiatry*, 30: 747–50.

Cochrane, R. (1992). Child abuse in Aboriginal families and its effects on the children's learning. *Early Child Development and Care*, 81: 131–36.

Cohen, D., Luchins, D., Eisdorfer, C., et al. (1990). Caring for relatives with Alzheimer's disease: The mental health risks to spouses, adult children, and other family caregivers. *Behavior, Health and Aging*, 1: 171–82.

Cohen, S., Hollingsworth, A., and Rubin, M. (1989). Another look at psychologic complications of hysterectomy. *Image: Journal of Nursing Scholarship*, 21: 51–3.

Cook, A., and Roy, R. (1995). Attitudes, beliefs, and illness behaviour. In R. Roy (Ed.), *Chronic pain in old age: An integrated biopsychosocial approach* (pp. 20–7). Toronto: University of Toronto Press.

Cook, A., and Thomas, M. (1994). Pain and use of health services among the elderly. *Journal of Aging Health*, 4: 155–72.

Crisp, R. (1996). Community integration, self-esteem, and vocational identity among persons with disabilities. *Australian Psychologist*, 31: 133–7.

Danoff-Burg, S., and Revenson, T. (2000). Rheumatic illness and relationships: Coping as a joint venture. In K. Schmaling, and T. Sher (Eds.), *The psychology of couples and illness: Theory, research and practice* (105–33). Washington, D.C.: American Psychological Association.

D'Arcy, C., and Siddique, C. (1987). Unemployment and health: An analysis of 'Canadian Health Survey' data. *International Journal of Health Services*, 15: 609–35.

Dell, P., and Papagiannidou, S. (1999). Hysterical talk? A discourse of Greek women's accounts of their experience following hysterectomy with oophorectomy. *Journal of Reproductive and Infant Psychology*, 17: 391–404.

Demlow, M., Liang, M., and Eaton, H. (1986). Impact of chronic arthritis in the elderly. *Clinics in Rheumatic Diseases*, 12: 329–35.

Derman, D. (2000). Grief and attachment in young widowhood. *Dissertation Abstracts International: Section A – Humanities and Social Sciences*, 60(7A): 2383.

deVries, B., Davis, C., Wortman, C., and Lehman, D. (1997). Long-term psychological and somatic consequences of later life parental bereavement. *Omega: Journal of Death and Dying*, 35: 97–117.

Dew, M., Penkower, L., and Bromet, E. (1991). Effects of unemployment on mental health in the contemporary family. *Behaviour Modification*, 15: 501–44.

Dowdy, S. (1999). Synchronous support, congruent coping, or a good marriage: Which is more important to the wife's perception of her husband's helpfulness in dealing with her rheumatoid arthritis pain? (Chronic Pain). *Dissertation Abstracts International: Section B – The Sciences and Engineering*, 60(6B): 2605.

Dozier, J. (1998). Lived experience of HIV-positive women. *Dissertation Abstracts International: Section A – Humanities and Social Sciences*, 58(11A): 4447.

Dunn, D. (1996). Well-being following amputation: Salutary effects of positive meaning, optimism, and control. *Rehabilitation Psychology*, 41: 285–302.

Dunn, K., Croft, P., and Hackett, G. (1999). Association of sexual problems with social, psychological, and physical problems in men and women: A cross-sectional population survey. *Journal of Epidemiology and Community Health*, 53: 144–8.

198 References

Dunning, P. (1993). Sexuality and women with diabetes. *Patient Education and Counseling*, 21: 5–14.

Dupuis, S. (1997) Understanding reproductive loss. *Dissertation Abstracts International: Section B – Sciences and Engineering*, 58(IN): 0414.

Eales, M. (1989). Shame among unemployed men. *Social Science and Medicine*, 28: 783–9.

Eisendrath, S., (1995). Psychiatric aspects of chronic pain. *Neuropathology*, 45: S26–S34.

Ellis-Hill, C., and Horn, S. (2000). Change in identity and self-concept: A new theoretical approach to recovery following a stroke. *Clinical Rehabilitation*, 14: 279–87.

Elliott, A., Smith, B., Penny, K., Smith, W., and Chambers, W. (1999). The epidemiology of chronic pain in the community. *Lancet*, 354: 1248–52.

El-Ruffaie, O., and Absood, G. (1993). Minor psychiatric morbidity in primary care: Prevalence, nature and severity. *International Journal of Social Psychiatry*, 7: 53–62.

Ernst, C. (1997). Epidemiology of depression in late life. *Current Opinion in Psychiatry*, 1: 107–12.

Ertekin, C. (1998). Diabetes mellitus and sexual dysfunction. *Scandinavian Journal of Sexology*, 1: 3–21.

Esplen, M.-J., Toner, B., Hunter, J., Glendon, G., Liede, A., Narod, S., Stuckless, N., Butler, K., and Field, B. (2000). A supportive-expressive group intervention for women with family history of breast cancer: Results of a Phase II study. *Psycho-Oncology*, 9 : 243–52.

Estlander, A., Takala, E., and Verkasalo, M. (1995). Assessment of depression in chronic musculoskeletal pain patients. *Clinical Journal of Pain*. 11: 194–200.

Fava, G., and Freyberger, H. (Eds.). *1998 Handbook of psychosomatic medicine*. Madison, Conn.: International Universities Press.

Ferrell, B.A., Ferrell, B.R., and Osterweil, D. (1990). Pain in the nursing home. *Journal of the American Geriatric Society*, 38: 401–4.

Ferrell, M., Gibson, S., and Helme, R. (1996). Chronic non-malignant pain in the elderly. In B. Ferrell and B.A. Ferrell (Eds.), *Pain in the elderly*. Seattle: IASP Press.

Ferroni, P.-A. (1994). Psychosexual sequelae of gynaecological conditions. *Sexual and Marital Therapy*, 9: 239–49.

Field, D., Minkler, M., Falk, F., and Leino, V. (1993). Influence of health on family contacts and family feelings in advanced old age: A longitudinal study. *Journal of Gerontology*, 48: 18–28.

Filiberti, A., Ripmonti, C., Totis, A., Ventafridda, V., De-Conno, F., Contiero, P., and Tamburin, M. (2001). Characteristics of terminal cancer patients who committed suicide during a home palliative care program. *Journal of Pain and Symptom Management*, 22: 544–53.

Fisher, B, Haythornthwaite, J., Heinberg, L., Clark, M., and Reed, J. (2001). Suicide intent in patients with chronic pain. *Pain*, 89: 199–206.

Fitzpatrick, T. (1998). Bereavement events among elderly men: The effects of stress and health. *Journal of Applied Gerontology*, 17: 204–28.

Flor, H., Turk, D., and Scholz, O. (1987). Impact of chronic pain on the spouse: Marital, emotional and physical consequences. *Journal of Psychosomatic Research*, 31: 63–72.

Fox, L., and Rau, M. (2001). Augmentative and alternative communication for adults following glossectomy and laryngectomy surgery. *AAC – Augmentative and Alternative Communication*, 17: 161–6.

Frank, E., Prigerson, H., Shear, M., and Reynolds, C. (1997). Phenomenology and treatment of bereavement related distress in the elderly. *International Clinical Psychopharmacology*, 12: S25–S29.

Freud, S. (1917). *Mourning and melancholia*. James Strachen, Ed. and Trans. Vol. 14 of The Standard Edition of the Psychological Works of Sigmund Freud. London: Hogarth 1973 (original ed. 1917).

Friedmann, M., and Webb, A. (1995). Family health and mental health six years after economic stress and unemployment. *Issues in Mental Health Nursing*, 16: 51–66.

Fukunishi, I. (1999). Relationship of cosmetic disfigurement to the severity of post-traumatic stress disorder in burn injury or digital amputation. *Psychotherapy and Psychosomatics*, 68: 82–6.

Gagliese, L., and Melzack, R. (1997). Chronic pain in elderly people. *Pain*, 70: 3–14.

Gallo, J., Royall, D., and Anthony, J. (1993). Risk factors for the onset of depression in middle age and later life. *Social Psychiatry and Psychiatric Epidemiology*, 28: 101–8.

Galyer, K., Conaglen, H., Hare, A., and Conaglen, J. (1999). The effect of gynaecological surgery on sexual desire. *Journal Sex and Marital Therapy*, 25: 81–8.

Gibson, S., and Helme, R. (1995). Age differences in pain perception and report: A review of physiological, laboratory and clinical studies. *Pain Reviews*, 2: 111–37.

Gilbar, O., and Eden, A. (2000–1). Suicide tendency in cancer patients. *Omega: Journal of Death and Dying*, 42: 159–70.

Goldsmith, A., Veum, J., and Darity, W. (1996). The impact of labour force history on self-esteem and its component parts, anxiety, alienation and depression. *Journal of Economic Psychology*, 17: 183–220.

Goochman, D. (Ed.). (1997). *Handbook of behaviour research: Personal and social determinants*. New York: Plenum.

Gurevich, M. (1998). Identity renegotiation in HIV positive women. *Dissertation Abstracts International: Section B – Sciences and Engineering*, 58(7B): 3967.

Halberg, L., and Carlsson, S. (1998). Psychosocial vulnerability and maintaining forces related to fibromyalgia: In-depth interviews with twenty-two female patients. *Scandinavian Journal of Caring Sciences*, 12: 95–103.

Hammarstroem, A., and Janlert, U. (1997). Nervous and depressive symptoms in a longitudinal study of youth unemployment – selection or exposure. *Journal of Adolescence*, 20: 293–305.

Hanisch, K. (1999). Job loss and unemployment research from 1994 to 1998: A review and recommendations for research and intervention. *Journal of Vocational Behavior*, 55: 188–220.

Harkins, S., Kwentus, J., and Price, D. (1984). Pain and the elderly. In C. Benedetti, C. Chapman, and G. Moricca (Eds.), *Advances in pain research and therapy* (pp. 103–21). New York: Raven Press.

Harvey, J. (1996). Preface. *Perspectus on loss*. Philadelphia: Brunner/Mazel.

Hayashi, T. (1994). Life review process in psychotherapy with the elderly. *Hiroshima Forum for Psychology*, 16: 53–63.

Heijmans, M., and De-Ridder, D. (1998). Structure and determinants of illness representations in chronic disease: A comparison of Addison's disease and chronic fatigue syndrome. *Journal of Health Psychology*, 3: 523–37.

Helson, R., and Wink, P. (1992). Personality change in women from the early 40's to the early 50's. *Psychology and Aging*, 7: 46–55.

Henriksson, M., Isometsa, E., Hietanen, S., Aro, H., and Lonnqvist, J. (1995). Mental disorders in cancer suicides. *Journal of Affective Disorders*, 36: 11–20.

Hitchcock, L., Ferrell, B., and McCaffery, M. (1994). The experience of chronic nonmalignant pain. *Journal of Pain and Symptom Management*, 5: 312–18.

Hoffman, W., Carpentier-Alting, P., Thomas, D., and Hamilton, V. (1991). Initial impact of plant closings on automobile workers and their families. *Families in Society*, 72: 103–7.

Hudgens, A. (1979). Family-oriented treatment of chronic pain. *Journal of Marriage Family Therapy*, 5: 67–78.

Hughes, D., and Kleepsies, P. (2001). Suicide in the mentally ill. *Suicide and Life Threatening Behavior*, 31(Suppl. 1): 48–59.

Jackson, T., Iezzi, A., and Lafreniere, K. (1997). The differential effects of employment status on chronic pain and healthy comparison groups. *International Journal of Behavioral Medicine*, 3: 354–69.

Jahoda, M., Lazarsfeld, P., and Zeisel, H. (1933). *Marienthal: The sociography of an unemployed community*. (English translation, 1971.) Chicago: Aldine-Atherton.

Jenson, S. (1985). Sexual dysfunction in female diabetics and alcoholics: A comparative study. *International Journal of Rehabilitation Research*, 8: 342–4.

– (1986). Sexual dysfunction in insulin-treated diabetics: A six-year follow-up study of 101 patients. *Archives of Sexual Behavior*, 15: 277–283.

Jex, S., Cvetanovski, J., and Allen, S. (1994). Self-esteem as a moderator of the impact of unemployment. *Journal of Social Behavior and Personality*, 9: 69–80.

Jones, L. (1990). Unemployment and child abuse. *Families in Society*, 71: 579–88.

– (1991). Unemployed fathers and their children: Implications for policy and practice. *Child and Adolescence Social Work Journal*, 8: 101–16.

Judd, D. (2001). 'To walk the last bit on my own' – narcissistic independence or identification with good objects: Issues of loss for a 13-year-old who had an amputation. *Journal of Child Psychotherapy*, 27: 47–67.

Karlawish, J., Casarett, D., Klocinski, J., and Clark, C. (2001). The relationship between caregivers' global ratings of Alzheimer's disease patients' quality of life, disease severity, and the caregiving experience. *Journal of American Geriatrics Society*, 8: 1066–70.

Katz, A. (1969). Wives of diabetic men. *Bulletin of the Menninger Clinic*, 33: 279–84.

Kav-Vennaki, S., and Zakham, L. (1983). Psychological effects of hysterectomy in premenopausal women. *Journal of Psychosomatic Obstetrics and Gynaecology*, 2: 76–80.

Keita, G., and Hurell, J. (Eds.). (1994). *Job stress in a changing workforce – investigating gender, diversity, and family issues*. Washington, D.C.: American Psychological Association.

Kelly, P. (1998). Loss experience in chronic pain and illness. In J. Harvey (Ed.), *Perspectives on loss: A sourcebook* (pp. 201–11). Philadelphia: Brunner/Mazel.

Kewman, D., and Tate, D. (1998). Suicide in SCI: A psychological autopsy. *Rehabilitation Psychology*, 43: 143–51.

Kissane, D., Block, S., McKenzie, M., McDowall, A., and Nitzan, R. (1998). Family grief therapy: A preliminary account of a new model to promote healthy family functioning during palliative care and bereavement. *Psychology Oncology*, 7: 14–25.

Kriegsman, D., Penninx, B., and van Eijk, T. (1994). Chronic disease in the elderly and its impact on the family: A review of the literature. *Family Systems Medicine*, 12: 249–67.

Kwentus, J., Harkins, S., Lignon, N., and Silverman, J. (1985). Current concepts of geriatric pain and its treatment. *Geriatrics*, 40: 48–57.

Kyriacou, D., Anglin, D., Taliaferro, E., Stone, S., Tubb, T., Linden, J., Muelleman, R., Barton, E., and Krause, J. (1999). Risk factors injury to women from domestic violence. *New England Journal of Medicine*, 341: 892–8.

Laatsch, L., and Shahani, B. (1996). The relationship between age, gender and psychological distress in rehabilitation in-patients. *Disability and Rehabilitation: An International Multidisciplinary Journal*, 18: 604–8.

Lalinec-Maced, M., and Englesmann, F. (1985). Anxiety, fears and depression related to hysterectomy. *Canadian Journal of Psychiatry*, 30: 44–7.

– (1988). Psychological profile of depresses women undergoing hysterectomy. *Journal of Psychosomatic Obstetrics and Gynaecology*, 8: 53–66.

Lalinec-Maced., M., Englesmann, F., and Marino, J. (1988). Depression and hysterectomy: A comparative study. *Psychosomatics*, 29: 307–14.

Lawrence, D., Almeida, O., Hulse, G., Jablensky, A., D'Arcy, C., and Holman, J. (2000). *Suicide and attempted suicide among older adults in Western Australia*. Cambridge: Cambridge University Press.

Leventhal, H., Idler, E., and Leventhal, E.A. (1999). The impact of chronic illness on the self system. In R. Contrada and R. Ashmore (Eds.), *Self, social identity, and physical health: Interdisciplinary explorations* (pp. 85–208). Vol. 2 of Rutgers Series on Self and Social Identity. 2. New York: Oxford University Press.

Lewis, G. (2001). Mental health after head injury. *Journal of Neurology, Neurosurgery and Psychiatry*, 71: 431.

Lewis, J. (1999). Status passages: The experience of HIV-positive gay men. *Journal of Homosexuality*, 37: 87–115.

Lieberman, M., and Fisher, L. (1995). The impact of chronic illness on the health and well-being of family members. *Gerontologist*, 35: 94–102.

Lobo, L., and Watkins, G. (1995). Late career unemployment in the 1990s: Its impact on the family. *Journal of Family Studies*, 1: 103–13.

Lower, N. (1995). Psychological adjustment with respect to cognitive and physical loss. *Dissertation Abstracts International: Section B – Sciences and Engineering*, 55(8B): 3593.

Lynch, M. (1995). The assessment and prevalence of affective disorders in advanced cancer. *Journal of Palliative Care*, 1: 10–18.

Maes, M., Calabrese, J., Lee, M., and Meltzer, H. (1994). Effects of age on spontaneous cortisolaemia of normal volunteers and depressed patients. *Psychoneuroendocrinology*, 19: 79–84.

Mahiacek, M. (1992). Logotherapy: A grief counseling process. *International Forum Logotherapy*, 5: 85–9.

Malkinson, R. (1996). Cognitive behavioral grief therapy. *Journal of Rational Emotive Cognitive Behavior Therapy*, 14: 155–71.

Mantyselka, P., Kumpusala, E., Ahonen, R., Kumpusalo, A., Kauhanen, J., Viinamaeki, H., Halogen, P., and Takala, J. (2001). Pain as a reason to visit the doctor: A study in Finnish primary health care. *Pain*, 89: 175–80.

Marotz-Baden, R., and Colvin, P. (1989). Adaptability, cohesion, and coping strategies of unemployed blue collar families with adolescents. *Lifestyles*, 10: 44–60.

Maruta, T., and Osborne, D. (1978). Sexual activity in chronic pain patients. *Psychosomatics*, 20: 241–8.

Mayer, M. (2001). Chronic sorrow in caregiving spouses of patients with Alzheimer's disease. *Journal of Aging and Identity*, 1: 49–60.

McCamish-Svensson, C., Samuelsson, G., Gillis, H., Svensson, T., and Dehlin, O. (1999). Social relationships and health as predictors of life satisfaction in advanced old age: Results from a Swedish longitudinal study. *International Journal of Aging and Human Development*, 48: 301–24.

McGuigan, J. (1995). Attributional style and depression in men receiving treatment for chronic pain. *Journal of Applied Rehabilitation and Counseling*, 26: 21–5.

Melanson, P., and Downe-Walmboldt, B. (1995). The stress of life with rheumatoid arthritis as perceived by older adults. *Activities, Adaptation and Aging*, 19: 33–47.

Melding, P. (1991). Is there such a thing as geriatric pain? *Pain*, 46: 119–21.

Meunier, G. (1994). Marital therapy with elderly couple. *Journal of Contemporary Psychotherapy*, 24: 125–9.

Miller, E., and Omarzu, J. (1998). New directions in loss research. In J. Harvey (Ed.), *Perspectives on loss: A sourcebook*. Philadelphia: Brunner/Mazel.

Mishara, B. (1999). Synthesis of research and evidence on factors affecting the desire of terminally ill person to hasten death. *Omega: Journal of Death and Dying*, 1: 1–70.

Mishra, S. (1992). Leisure activities and life satisfaction in old age: A case study of retired government employees living in urban areas. *Activities and Adaptation*, 16: 7–16.

Monahan, D., and Hooker, K. (1995). Health of spouse caregivers of dementia patients: The role of personality and social support. *Social Work*, 40: 305–14.

Monga, T., Monga, U., Tan, G., and Grabois, M. (1999). Coital positions and sexual functioning in patients with chronic pain. *Sexuality and Disability*, 17: 287–97.

Monga, T., Tan, G., Ostermann, H., Monga, U., and Grabois, M. (1998). Sexuality and sexual adjustment of patients with chronic pain. *Disability and Rehabilitation – An International Multidisciplinary Journal*, 20: 317–29.

Montenero, P., and Donatone, E. (1962). Diabète et activité sexuelle chez l'homme. *Diabète*, 10: 327–35.

Moss, M., Lawton, M., and Glicksman, A. (1991). The role of pain in the last year of life in the older person. *Journal of Gerontology*, 42: 51–7.

Nau, D. (1997). Andy writes to his amputated leg: Utilizing letter writing as an interventive technique of family grief therapy. *Journal of Family Psychotherapy*, 8: 1–12.

Neimeyer, R. (1999). Narrative strategies in grief therapy. *Journal of Constructivist Psychology*, 12: 65–85.

Newman, A., and Bertelson, A. (1986). Sexual dysfunction in diabetic women. *Journal of Behavioral Medicine*, 9: 261–70.

Nord, D. (1997). Threats to identity in survivors of multiple AIDS-related losses. *American Journal of Psychotherapy*, 3: 387–402.

Oriol, W. (1991). Chronic pain. *Perspective on Aging*, 20: 6–13.

Pain and Aging. (2001). Special issue. *Pain Research and Management*, 3: 116–65.

Parkes, M. (1973). *Bereavement: Studies of grief in adult life*. Harmondsworth: Penguin.

Parkes, M., and Weiss, R. (1983). *Recovery from bereavement*. New York: Basic Books.

Parmelee, P., Katz, I., and Lawton, M. (1991). The relation of pain to depression among institutionalized aged. *Journal of Gerontology: Psychological Sciences*, 46: 15–21.

Peters, A., and Liefbroer, A. (1997). Beyond marital status: Partner history and well-being in old age. *Journal of Marriage and the Family*, 59: 687–99.

Peterson, Y. (1979). The impact of physical disability on marital adjustment: A literature review. *Family Coordinator*, 28: 47–51.

Poole, J. (2000). Habits in women with chronic disease: A pilot study. *Occupational Therapy Journal of Research*, 20: 112S–118S.

Price, R. (1992). Psychosocial impact of job loss on individuals and families. *Current Directions in Psychological Science*, 1: 9–11.

Price, R., Friedland, D., and Vinokur, A. (1996). Job loss: Hard times and eroded identity. In J. Harvey (Ed.), *Perspectives on loss: A sourcebook* (pp. 303–16). Philadelphia: Brunner/Mazel.

Prigerson, H., Maciejewski, P., and Rosenheck, R. (1999). The effects of marital dissolution and marital quality on heath and health service use among women. *Medical Care*, 37: 858–73.

– (2000). Preliminary explorations of the harmful interactive effects of widowhood and marital harmony on health, health service use, and health care costs. *Gerontologist*, 40: 349–57.

Pruchno, R., and Potashnik, S. (1989). Caregiving spouses: Physical and mental health in perspective. *Journal of the American Geriatric Society*, 37: 697–705.

Pruchno, R., Kleban, M., Michaels, J., and Dempsey, N. (1990). Mental and physical health of caregiving spouses: Development of a causal model. *Journal of Gerontology*, 45: 192–9.

Psoralea, H., and Adela, A. (1992). The prevalence and context of family violence against children in Finland. *Child Abuse and Neglect*, 16: 823–32.

Randolph, J., Arnett, P., Higginson, C., and Williams, D. (2000). Neurovegetative symptoms in multiple sclerosis: Relationship to depressed mood, fatigue, and physical disability. *Archives of Clinical Neuropsychology*, 15: 387–98.

Raphael, B. (1982). *The anatomy of bereavement*. New York: Basic Books.

Rask, N. (1978). Quality of life and factors affecting the response to hysterectomy. *Journal of Family Practice*, 7: 483–8.

Reed, L. (1999). The efficacy of grief therapy as a treatment modality for individuals diagnosed with co-morbid disorders of chronic pain and depression. *Dissertation Abstracts International: Section B – Sciences and Engineering*, 59(7B): 3710.

Reisine, S. (1995). Arthritis and the family. *Arthritis Care and Research*, 8: 265–71.

Reisine, S., and Fifield, J. (1995). Family work demands, employment demands, and depressive symptoms in women with rheumatoid arthritis. *Women and Health*, 22: 25–45.

Rethelyi, J., Berghammer, R., and Kopp, M. (2001). Comorbidity of pain-associated disability and depressive symptoms in connection with sociodemographic variables: results from a cross-sectional epidemiological survey in Hungary. *Pain*, 93: 115–21.

Roeske, N. (1978). Quality of life and factors affecting the response to hysterectomy. *Journal of Family Practice* 7: 483–8.

Rooparinesingh, S., and Gopeesingh, T. (1982). Hysterectomy and its psychological aftermath. *West Indian Medical Journal*, 31: 131–4.

Rose, M. (1997). Sexuality and chronic illness: A biopsychocial model of sexual satisfaction in women with interstitial cystitis. *Dissertation Abstracts: International: Section B – Sciences and Engineering*, 57(10B): 6591.

Rossi, A. (Ed). (1994). *Sexuality across the life course.* Chicago: University of Chicago Press.

Rowe, J., and Besdine, R. (Eds.). (1982). *Health and disease in old age.* Boston: Little Brown.

Roy, R. (1989). *Chronic pain and the family. A problem-centered perspective.* New York: Human Sciences Press (Plenum).

– (1998). *Childhood abuse and chronic pain: A curious relationship.* Toronto: University of Toronto Press.

– (2001). *Chronic pain and social relations.* New York: Kluwer/Plenum.

Roy, R. and Thomas, M. (1986). A survey of chronic pain in an elderly population. *Canadian Family Physician*, 31: 513–16.

– (1987). Elderly persons with and without pain, part 1. *Clinical Journal of Pain*, 3: 102–6.

– (1988). Pain, depression and illness behavior in a group of community-based elderly persons: Elderly persons with and without pain, part 2. *Clinical Journal of Pain*, 3: 207–11.

Roy, R., Thomas, K., and Berger, S. (1990). A comparative study of Canadian non-clinical and British pain clinic subjects. *Clinical Journal of Pain*, 3: 213–22.

Rubin, A., and Babbott, D. (1958). Impotence and diabetes mellitus. *Journal of the American Medical Association*, 168: 498–500.

Rubin, S., and Schechter, N. (1997). Exploring the social construction of bereavement: Perceptions of adjustment and recovery in bereaved men. *American Journal of Orthopsychiatry*, 67: 279–89.

Rumzek, H. (1998). Does unemployment become a major stressor in the evolution of chronic pain? *Dissertation Abstracts International: Section B – Sciences and Engineering*, 58(7B): 3914.

Ruoff, G. (1996). Depression in the patient with chronic pain. *Journal of Family Practice*, 43: S25–S34.

Ruskin, P. (1985). Geropsychiatric consultation in a university hospital: A report on 67 referrals. *American Journal of Psychiatry*, 142: 333–6.

Scharloo, M., Kaptein, A., Weinman, J., Hazes, J., Willems, L., Bergman, W., and Rooijmans, H. (1998). Illness perceptions, coping and functioning in patients with rheumatoid arthritis, chronic pulmonary disease and psoriasis. *Journal of Psychosomatic Research*, 5: 573–85.

Schliebner, C., and Peregoy, J. (1994). Unemployment effects on the family and the child: Interventions for counselors. *Journal of Counseling and Development*, 72: 368–72.

Schoffling, K. (1963). Disorders of sexual functions in male diabetics. *Diabetes*, 12: 519–27.

Schulz, R., and Scott, B. (1999). Caregiving as a risk factor for mortality: The caregiver health effect study. *Journal of the American Medical Association*, 282: 1–9.

Sengstaken, E., and King, S. (1993). The problems of pain and its detection among geriatric nursing home residents. *Journal of the American Geriatric Society*, 41: 541–4.

Shanas, E. (1979). National survey of the elderly: Report to administration on aging. Washington, D.C.: Department of Health and Human Services.

Shanks-McElroy, H., and Strobino, J. (2001). Male caregivers of spouses with Alzheimer's disease: Risk factors and health status. *American Journal of Alzheimer's Disease*, 3: 167–75.

Shapiro, E. (1994). *Grief as a family process: A developmental approach to clinical practice*. New York: Guilford.

Sheeran, P., Abrams, D., and Orbell, S. (1995). Unemployment, self-esteem, depression: A social comparison theory. *Basic and Applied Social Psychology*, 17: 65–82.

Stang, P., Von Korff, M., and Galer, B. (1998). Reduced labour force participation among primary care patients with headache. *Journal of General Internal Medicine*, 13: 296–302.

Starkey, J. (1996). Race differences in the effect of unemployment on marital instability: A socioeconomic analysis. *Journal of Socio-Economics*, 25: 683–720.

Steiner, M., and Aleksandrowicz, D. (1970). Psychiatric sequelae to gynaecological operations. *Israel Annals of Psychiatry and Related Disciplines*, 8: 186–92.

Sternbach, R. (1986). Survey of pain in the United States: The Nuprin Pain Report. *Clinical Journal of Pain*, 2: 49–53.

Stoller, E., and Forster, L. (1994). The impact of symptom interpretation of physician utilization, *Journal of Aging and Health*, 6: 507–34.

Stratton, K., Maisick, R., Wrigley, J., White, M., Johnson, P., and Fine, P. (1996). Barriers to return to work among persons unemployed due to arthritis and musculoskeletal disorders. *Arthritis and Rheumatism*, 39: 101–9.

Strauss, A. and Corbi, J. (Eds.). (1997). *Ground theory in practice*. Thousand Oaks, Calif.: Sage.

Stroebe, M. (1992). Coping with bereavement: A review of the grief work hypothesis. *Omega: Journal of Death and Dying*, 26:19–42.

Stroebe, M., Schut, H., and Stroebe W. (1998). Trauma and grief: A comparative analysis. In J. Harvey (Ed.), *Perspectives on loss: A sourcebook* (pp. 81–94). Philadelphia: Brunner/Mazel.

Suris, J., Parera, N., Puig, C. (1996). Chronic illness and emotional distress. *Journal of Adolescent Health*, 19: 153–6.

Swensen, C., and Fuller, S. (1992). Expression of love, marriage problems, commitment, and anticipatory grief in the marriages of cancer patients. *Journal of Marriage and the Family*, 54: 191–6.

Tan, G., Monga, U., Thornby, J., and Monga, T. (1998). Sexual functioning, age, and depression revisited. *Sexuality and Disability*, 16: 77–86.

Tebb, S., and Jivanjee, P. (2000). Caregiver isolation: An ecological model. *Journal of Gerontological Social Work*, 2: 51–72.

Tewksbury, R., and McGaughey, D. (1998). Identities and identity transformations among persons with HIV disease. *Journal of Gay, Lesbian, and Bisexual Identity*, 3: 213–32.

Thomas, M., and Roy, R. (1999). *The changing nature of pain complaints over the life span*. New York: Plenum.

Thompson, S. (1998). Blockades to finding meaning and control. In J. Harvey (Ed)., *Perspectives on loss: A source book* (pp. 21–34). Philadelphia: Brunner/Mazel.

Thompson, S., and Kyle, D. (2000). The role of perceived control in coping with the losses associated with chronic illness. In J. Harvey and E. Miller (Eds.), *Loss and trauma: general and close relationships perspectives* (pp. 131–45). New York: Brunner Routledge, Taylor and Francis Group.

Tunks, E., and Roy, R. (1982). Chronic pain and the occupational role. In R. Roy and E. Tunks (Eds.), *Chronic pain: Psychosocial factors in rehabilitation* (pp. 53–67). Baltimore, MD: Williams and Wilkins.

Turpin, T., and Heath, D. (1979). The link between hysterectomy and depression. *Canadian Journal of Psychiatry*, 24: 247–54.

Vali, F., and Walkup, J. (1998). Combined medical and psychological symptoms: Impact on disability and health care utilization of patients with arthritis. *Medical Care*, 36: 1073–84.

Valkenberg, H. (1988). Epidemiologic considerations of the geriatric population. *Gerontology*, 34 (Suppl): 2–10.

van Grootheest, D., Beckman, A., van Groenou, M., Broesse, M., and Deeg, D. (1999). Sex differences in depression after widowhood: Do men suffer more? *Social Psychiatry and Psychiatric Epidemiology*, 34: 391–8.

Verma, S., and Gallagher, R. (2000). Evaluating and treating, co-morbid pain and depression. *International Review of Psychiatry*, 12: 103–14.

Viinamaeki, H., Koskela, K., and Niskanen, L. (1996). Rapidly declining mental well-being during unemployment. *European Journal of Psychiatry*, 10: 215–21.

Vilhjalmsson, R., Kristjansdottir, G., and Sveinbjarnardottir, E. (1998). Factors associated with suicide ideation in adults. *Social Psychiatry and Psychiatric Epidemiology*, 3: 97–103.

Vitaliano, P., Scanlan, J., Krenz, C., et al. (1996). Psychological distress, caregiving, and metabolic variables. *Journals of Gerontology: Series B – Psychological Sciences and Social Sciences*, 51: 290–9.

Von Korff, M., Ormel, J., Keefe, F., and Dworkin, S. (1992). Grading the severity of chronic pain. *Pain*, 50: 133–49.

Wade, T. (1999). Stress and distress among husbands and wives. *Dissertation Abstracts International: Section A – Humanities and Social Sciences*, 59(7A): 2736.

Weiss, R. (1998). Issues in the study of loss and grief. In J. Harvey (Ed.), *Perspectives of Loss: A Sourcebook* (pp. 343–51). Philadelphia: Brunner/Mazel.

Whitley, D., Beck, E., and Rutowski, R. (1989). Cohesion and organisation patterns among family members coping with rheumatoid arthritis. *Social Work in Health Care*, 29: 79–95.

Whitley-Reed, L. (1999). The efficacy of grief therapy as a treatment modality for individuals diagnosed with co-morbid disorders of chronic pain and depression. *Dissertation Abstracts International: Section B – Sciences and Engineering*, 59(7B): 3710.

Williams, A. (1998). Depression in chronic pain: Mistaken models, missed opportunities. *Scandinavian Journal of Behaviour Therapy*, 27: 61–80.

Williamson, G., Schulz, R., Bridges, M., and Behan, A. (1984). Social and psychological factors in adjustment to limb amputation. *Journal of Social Behavior and Personality*, 9: 249–68.

Willmott, M., and Broome, A. (Ed.). (1989). *Health psychology: Process and applications*. London: Chapman and Hall.

Winokuer, H. (2000). The impact of expected versus unexpected death on the surviving spouse. *Dissertation Abstracts International: Section B – Sciences and Engineering*, 61(1B): 553.

Worden, J. (1991). *Grief counseling and grief therapy: A handbook for the mental health practitioner* (2nd ed.). New York: Springer-Verlag.

Wortman, C., and Silver, R. (1989). The myths of coping with loss. *Journal of Clinical and Consulting Psychology*, 57: 349–57.

Xu, H., Xiao, S., Chen, J., and Liu, L. (2000). Epidemiological study on committed suicide among the elderly in some urban and rural areas of Hunan province, China. *Chinese Mental Health Journal*, 2: 121–4.

Yee, J., and Schulz, R. (2000). Gender differences in psychiatric morbidity among family caregivers: A review and analysis. *Gerontologist*, 40: 147–64.

Zautra, A., Hamilton, N., and Burke, H. (1999). Comparison of stress responses in women with two types of chronic pain: Fibromyalgia and osteoarthritis. *Cognitive Therapy and Research*, 23: 209–30.

Index

abandonment, feelings of, 29, 32, 34, 55, 120, 179

abdominal pain, 91–3, 113, 118, 181

Abraido-Lanza, A.-F., 66

Abrams, D., 50

Absood, G., 105

abuse, 120, 160, 162, 163; of a child, 24, 51–2, 151, 160–3; of a partner, 52, 116, 117, 122, 158

acceptance, of loss, 5, 33, 41, 47, 58, 136, 137, 138, 141, 165, 168, 172, 179, 183, 186, 187, 189

activities of daily living, 63, 141, 166. *See also* residual activities

acute illness, 62

adolescent, 63, 119, 144, 145, 177, 183

adoption, 36

affective roles, 87

African-American women study, 13

age, 4, 8–9, 13, 18–19, 24, 31, 58, 89–90, 93–4, 103–6, 111, 112, 113–16, 119, 124–6, 128–9, 131, 134, 138, 149, 174; and attitude to pain, 127, 141, 187; and suicide, 143–5; when widowed, 33

ageism, 141

AIDS, 70–2

Akechi, T., 149

alarm reaction, 5, 34

alcoholism, 24, 36, 44, 51, 54, 116–18, 119–21, 147

Aleksandrowicz, D., 14

alienation, feelings of, 10, 69. *See also* isolation; loneliness

Allebeck, P., 148, 150

Allen, S. 49

Allumbaugh, D., 137, 168–9

Almgren, G., 52

Alonzo, A., 26

Alzheimer's disease, 125–6, 131–3, 166

Amir, M., 150

amputation, 5–12, 165, 169, 171, 187. *See also* hysterectomy; loss of limb; phantom limb

Amputation Study, 5

analgesics, 30

Ananth, J., 14

Andelman, F., 144–5

Anderson, B., 14

Anderson, H., 128
anger, 11, 29, 32, 34, 58, 64, 69, 83, 85, 96, 99, 100, 102, 120, 123, 134, 154, 155, 156, 159, 180; and suicide, 150
anorexia, 59, 121
Anthony, J., 106
anti-hypertensive drugs, 103
anti-social activity, 88, 100, 178
antidepressants, 28, 32, 36, 41, 85, 158–9
anxiety, 5, 6, 11, 30, 34, 49, 65, 79, 95, 105, 109, 134, 181, 182
appetite, loss of, 6, 136
Arab studies, 105
Archer, J., 46
Arluke, A., 74
arthritis. *See* rheumatoid arthritis
assessment: of depression, 21, 49, 148, 151; of family, 84; of hopelessness, 148; of mental status, 164. *See also* psychiatric assessment; psychosocial assessment
asthma, 145
attachment, separation, and loss, 3
atypical grief, 24–6, 31, 73, 136–8, 188–9
Australian studies, 52, 70, 149–50
automobile accident, 28, 29, 35–6, 44, 50–1, 58, 96, 97, 98, 153–4, 156, 159, 160–2
Averill, P., 48

Babbott, D., 111
back pain, 72, 78, 83, 88, 93–4, 120, 138, 159, 190; and credibility, 45; and employment, 35–6, 59–60, 72,

118; and old age, 125–6, 128; and sexual function, 111; and suicide, 150
bankruptcy, 51, 96
Banks, S., 107
Barbato, A., 137
Barling, J., 53
Barlow, J., 83
Barron, W., 151
Bartos, M., 70
battery, 188
Beck Depression Inventory, 21, 49, 148, 151
Beck Hopelessness Scale, 148
Bedard, M., 132
behavioural therapy, 158–9, 169, 180
Bengesser, G., 157
Bennett, K., 34
bereavement, 3, 4, 5, 6, 15, 34, 137–8, 165, 167, 184, 189, 190
Berger, S., 128
Berghammer, R., 108
Bernhard, L., 13–14
Bertelson, A., 109
Besdine, R., 128
betrayal, 32, 34, 90–1
Bhatia, M., 16–17
Bhojak, M., 10
biological factors, 25, 151
Bjorndal, A., 47–8
Blake, D., 110
Bleich, C., 53
blindness, 188
body image, 10, 14, 151, 170, 182
Bolund, C., 148, 150
bone disease, 128
Bonnanno, G., 140

boundaries, 69, 71, 180

Bouras, N., 110

Bowlby, J., 3–4, 7, 19, 21, 136, 169

brain hemorrhage, 126, 134

brain cancer, 145

Brauhn, N.E.H., 70

breadwinner, 44, 69, 83, 87, 98. *See also* family roles; financial circumstances

breast cancer 125, 129, 133

Bridges, P., 110

Bromberger, J., 105

Bromet, E., 53

Bruce, M., 26

burden to others, 142, 146

burn injury, 8

Buttenshaw, P., 171

Cacioppo, J., 133

cancer, 18, 93–4, 125–6, 128–9, 134, 138, 142, 164; and grief therapy, 166, 171; and suicide, 145–50

capital punishment, 69

cardiac problem, 91

caregivers, 125, 131–4

caretaker, 89. *See also* family roles

Carlsson, S., 24

Carnelley, K., 34

Carr, D., 30–1

case studies: Mr Abrams, 10–11, 23; Mr Bassett, 11–12; Mrs Cliff, 17–18; Mrs Davies, 28–34, 42, 176–81; Mrs Eric, 35–8; Mr Frum, 38–9, 42; Ms. Gill, 39–42; Mr Hill, 54–6; Mrs Innes, 56–8, 63–8, 79–80, 172–6, 184–5; Mr James, 58–60, 153–7, 164; Mr Kelly, 72–7, 80–1; Mrs

Lynn, 85–91, 100–1; Mr Morton, 91–3, 101–2; Mrs Neil, 93–6, 103; Mr Oscar, 96–101; Ms. Peters, 113–16, 181–5; Ms. Quill, 116–18, 121–2; Mr Roper, 118–20; Mrs Semple, 120–2; Mrs Thomas, 125–6, 129, 131, 133–8, 166; Ms. Una, 138–41; Mr Vince, 157–60, 164

catharsis, 136, 137, 165

cerebrovascular accident, 9

Charmaz, K, 65, 69, 75, 80–1

chemotherapy, 147

chest pain, 35

Chicago studies, 52

child abuse, 24, 51–2, 151, 160–3

childhood, 24, 30, 37, 40, 63, 73, 91, 93, 116, 119, 123, 151, 162, 163, 176

children, and responsibilities for, 3, 4, 13, 29, 30, 32, 34, 36, 37, 38, 40, 44, 58, 67, 68, 71, 73, 75, 76, 80, 81, 85, 86, 88–91, 94, 96, 98–101, 114–16, 119–21, 125, 126, 129, 134, 135, 146, 153, 156–8, 161, 175, 177, 178, 182, 184

Chinese studies, 144

Christoffersen, M., 51, 53–4

chronic illness, 15, 21, 22, 23, 37, 41, 42, 44, 47, 54, 60, 65, 67, 69, 72, 75, 79, 80, 83, 84, 96, 101, 102, 103ff, 110, 112, 122, 124, 132, 133, 137, 141, 142, 144, 145, 153, 165, 170, 171, 175, 183, 184–6, 188, 190–1; and depression, 24–8, 108–9; and identity, 73–4, 77–8, 91–3; and suicide, 143–5

chronic pain, 21, 26, 43, 58, 72, 76, 81, 86, 104, 125–9, 130, 131, 142,

148, 170; and depression, 28, 105–
8, 124, 152; and grief therapy, 184–
5, 190–1; onset of, 58; and
progression of losses, 22–3, 37;
sexual function and, 38, 111–13,
122–3, 174; and suicide, 150–3;
unpredictability of, 41–2, 65–6
chronic sick role, 62, 74, 75, 77, 82,
179, 191
Ciaramella, A., 146
Clark, W., 53–4
class, social, 51. *See also* blue-collar
workers; white-collar workers
Claussen, B., 47–8
Clayton, P., 34
client-centred therapy, 168, 171
Cochrane, R., 52
cognitive therapy, 136, 158, 169, 180
Cohen, D., 133
Colvin, P., 53
competence, 66
computer-assisted tomographic
(CAT) scan, 125
conflictual relationships, 25, 30–1,
34–5
confusion, 96, 97, 125, 183
congenital hip problem, 120
conjugal role, 173–4. *See also*
marriage; sexual function
control, 10, 27, 94–5, 180; loss of,
45–7, 149, 164, 172–6; restoration
of, 170
Cook, A., 127
coping styles, 137, 143, 150, 165, 167;
and gender, 71–2
cortisol levels, 105
couples therapy, 171

courage, 127
credibility, of patient, 45, 69
criminal activity, 44, 51, 88
crisis theories, 33
Croft, P., 109
cultural beliefs, 31, 137, 164
Cvetanovski, J., 49
cystitis, interstitial, 112

D'Arcy, C., 43
danazol, 17
Danish studies, 51
Danoff-Burg, S., 83
Darity, W., 50
death, 3, 4, 5, 7, 52, 123, 139, 146,
165, 167, 169, 171, 187; of a child,
125, 126, 134–8, 166; of a husband,
24, 28–35, 39–45, 179–9, 181; of a
mother, 105, 140, 141, 143, 176; of
a parent, 7, 8, 30; of a spouse, 7,
25, 124, 188; sudden, 28–9, 31, 34–
5, 125–6, 134, 166
decathexis, 167
defence mechanism, 10, 11, 57, 58
delayed grief, 24, 136
Dell, P., 13
Demlow, M., 128
denial, 5, 11–12, 63, 77, 121, 165
depression, 9, 10, 15, 16, 18, 21, 24,
26, 34, 37, 41, 44, 69, 83, 86, 87, 99,
100, 103, 105, 115, 124, 133, 134,
137, 139, 142, 143, 144, 151, 153,
162, 163, 164, 168, 188, 191; and
cancer, 145–50; and chronic pain,
106–8, 152; and grief therapy, 170–
1, 190; and multiple stresses, 76–7,
85, 88, 98; and rheumatoid

arthritis, 27, 39–40; and sexual function, 38, 111–13, 122–3, 174; and unemployment, 48–9, 51, 58–9, 61

depression-disability relationship, 26

depression-suicide relationship, 152

Derman, D., 33

despair, 46, 166, 174

deVries, B., 135

Dew, M., 53

diabetes, 11, 103, 109, 110, 122, 189

diagnostic issues, 108, 138–9, 190

Diagnostic and Statistical Manual of Mental Disorders (DSM), 146–7

diet, 94

disability, 10, 27, 37, 59, 60, 63, 73, 75, 77, 78, 79, 83, 89, 96, 102, 103, 129, 140, 142, 143, 149, 152, 153, 161–3, 165, 166, 170, 191

disequilibirium, state of, 168

disfigurement, 8, 69

divorce, 37, 73, 95, 117, 119

domestic roles, 38, 173

Donatone, E., 111

Dowdy, S., 83

Downe-Walmboldt, B., 128

Dozier, J., 71

drugs, illicit, 116, 117, 152, 154

DSM. *See Diagnostic and Statistical Manual of Mental Disorders*

Dunn, D., 10

Dunn, K., 109

Dupuis, S., 12–13, 18

Dutch studies, 130

dying, 45, 165

dyspareunia, 109

dysthymia, 99

Eaton, H., 128

ecological system (patient's), 82

Eden, A., 147–8

education, 16, 31, 52–3, 94, 105, 106, 117–18; and recovery, 13–14

ego-oriented therapy, 136

Eisendrath, S., 107

El-Ruffaie, O., 105

elderly patients, 3, 124, 125, 127–8, 130–1, 139, 141, 145, 165, 171, 187; and suicide, 143–4

Elliott, A., 126

Ellis-Hill, C., 27

emotional consequences of pain, 168

employment, 26, 35–6, 43–4, 45, 48–54, 58–9, 61, 69, 72, 85, 118; and loss of roles, 26, 47, 56–7, 68–9, 172–3, 187–8; and self-esteem, 45–7, 49–50, 66. *See also* job loss; work

empty nest syndrome, 106

endometriosis, 17, 116, 117, 123

Englesmann, F., 16, 18

epidemiology, 143

epilepsy, 144

erectile problems, 109

Ernst, C., 143–4

Ertekin, C., 109

Esplen, M.-J., 171

Estlander, A., 108

existentialism, and loss, 124, 142, 146

expectations, 17, 20, 67, 75, 82, 83, 96, 154, 156, 159, 176; of medical procedures, 9–10, 17–18, 20, 73, 153; patient's family's, 92–4

family, 31, 32, 36, 38, 44, 52–3, 59, 61, 63, 68, 73, 80, 82ff, 92, 105, 115,

123, 129, 132, 137, 139, 154, 156, 157, 158, 160, 164, 168, 170, 172, 178, 180, 181, 183, 187; roles, 39, 51, 66–7, 89–90, 93–102, 111, 125–6, 130–1, 134, 138, 177–9; violence, 44, 52–3, 60, 126. *See also,* children; father; husband; mother; wife

Family Assessment Device, 84
Family Assessment Measure, 84
family therapy, 83, 131, 136, 171
fatalistic attitude, 127
father, and fathering, 31, 51, 55, 69, 85, 89, 97, 98, 116, 126, 133, 154, 176, 178, 180
fatigue, 27
fear, 5, 11, 34, 40, 57, 95, 121, 146, 157–8
Ferrell, B.A., 128, 150–1
Ferrell, B.R., 128
Ferrell, M., 128
Ferroni, P.-A., 18
fertility (reproductive) issues, 113–16, 118, 123, 181–5
fibromyalgia, 24, 26, 93, 150
Field, D., 130
Fifield, J., 83
Filiberti, A., 146
financial situation, 36–8, 40, 56, 60, 72, 75, 76, 83, 94, 96, 107, 122, 124, 126, 135, 144, 150, 154, 157, 161, 166, 180; control over, 97–8; and family violence, 52–3
Finnish studies, 51–2, 108
Fisher, B., 151
Fisher, L., 133
Fitzpatrick, T., 135

Flor, H., 111
Forster, L., 127
Fox, L., 171
Frank, E., 137
Freud, S., 21, 168
Friedland, D., 44
Friedmann, M., 53
friend, 8, 38, 62, 73, 78, 105, 114, 117, 124, 130, 139, 145, 173, 180, 182
frustration, 99
Fukunishi, I., 8
Fuller, S. 171
functions, 25, 172, 191

Gagliese, L., 127
Galer, B., 43
Gallagher, R., 27
Gallo, J., 106
Galyer, K., 18
gastritis, 55, 72
gay community, 70
gender issues, 8–9, 14, 24, 49, 51, 71–2, 89, 93, 95–6, 101, 105, 109–10, 128, 130–1, 133, 145, 154
genetic factors, 151
geriatric pain patients. *See* elderly patients
geropsychiatric service, 131
Gestalt therapy, 168–9
Gibson, S., 128
Gilbar, O., 147–8
Glickman, A., 105, 128
goals, 81, 139, 70, 172, 175, 179, 190
Goldsmith, A., 50
Gopeesingh, T., 14
grief, 3–5, 9, 18, 19, 21, 23, 24, 25, 26, 27, 28, 31, 34, 37, 38, 41, 61, 68,

106, 115, 135, 137, 138, 141, 171,
183, 185; and loss of control, 172–
6; and loss of roles, 45–7 and
passim; not equivalent to depression, 190; stages of, 22, 33, 39, 136,
165, 166, 187
grief determinants. *See* theory of
grief
grieving process: conceptual
framework for, 3–4; for other than
death, 58, 166, 187–91; and
depression, 190; length of, 33; and
loss of wife or loss of limb, 7t;
'normal,' 15, 19; and unemployment, 26; and unpredictability of
chronic pain, 41–2, 65–6
group therapy, 180–1
guilt, 24, 30, 31, 47, 71, 83, 86, 88,
100, 115, 116, 117–18, 123, 134,
162, 168, 173, 181
Gurevich, M., 71
Guthrie, E., 109

Hackett, G., 109
Halberg, L., 24
Hamilton Depression Rating Scale,
146–7
Hamilton, N., 24
Hammarstroem, A., 48
Hanisch, K., 53
Harkins, S., 126
Harvey, J., 7–8
Hayashi, T., 171
headache, 28–34, 36, 79, 83–5,
89, 111, 120, 124, 138, 157,
158–60, 177, 178, 179. *See also*
migraine

health, loss of, 3, 7, 9, 21, 25, 37,
42, 65, 80; may or may not be
irretrievable, 169
heart: attack, 31, 95, 178; disease,
103, 110
Heath, D., 16
Helme, R., 128
helplessness, 37, 39, 87, 97, 99, 162,
164
helplessness-depression link, 164
Helson, R., 106
Henriksson, M., 147–50
herpes zoster, 80, 128
hip problems, 120
Hitchcock, L. 150–1
HIV, 70–2
Hjort, P., 47–8
Hoffman, W., 53
homicide, 52
Hooker, K., 133
hope, 65, 174
hopelessness, 24, 27, 39, 51, 97, 99,
124, 143, 148, 149, 156, 157, 163,
164, 190; assessment of, 148; and
grief therapy, 179
Horn, S., 27
household responsibilities, 94, 173,
177
Hoyt, W., 137, 168–9
Hudgens, A., 111
Hughes, D., 145
humiliation, 52, 76, 121, 156, 175, 188
humour, 170
Hungarian studies, 108
husband, and role of, 59, 75, 76, 85,
86, 87, 88, 89, 90, 91, 93, 95, 96, 97,
98, 99, 100, 102, 121, 125, 126, 129,

131, 133, 138, 154, 158, 162, 173, 174, 176, 177, 180; death of, 28–35, 178–9, 181

hypochondriasis, 107

hypothalamic-pituitary-adrenal axis, 105

hysterectomy, 8, 12, 13, 14, 15–20, 113–15, 123, 181

Icelandic studies, 108, 144, 157

identity, 13, 14, 18, 63, 69, 70, 71, 72, 73, 75, 77, 78, 79, 83, 99, 114, 115, 140, 157, 158, 162, 168, 170, 181, 187, 191; and grief therapy, 172–6; loss of and suicide, 153; preservation of, 80–1; redefinition of, 39, 42, 64–8, 80–1, 166–7, 185

Idler, E., 67

Iezzi, A., 43

immigration, 60, 93–4, 113, 119, 153

immune response, 133

impotence, 189

Indian studies, 16–17, 130

individualized outcomes, 4, 26, 102, 150, 190

insurance companies, 75, 161–2

intellectual recognition of loss, 137, 165

intervention strategies, 166, 191. *See also various therapies and treatments*

invalid status, 39, 42, 139

irretrievable losses, 169, 172

irritable bowel syndrome, 78

Irwin, H., 137

isolation, feelings of, 31, 97, 113–14, 123, 140, 143. *See also* alienation

Israeli Index of Potential Suicide (IIPSE), 147–8

Jackson, T., 43

Jahoda, M., 45

Janlert, U., 48

Jenson, S., 110

Jex, S., 49

Jivanjee, P., 132

job loss, 84, 172, 187–8. *See also* employment; work

joint pain, 64, 67, 124, 128, 129

Jones, L., 53

Judd, D., 171

Karlawish, J., 132

Katz, A., 111

Katz, I., 128

Kav-Vennaki, S., 16

Kelly, P. 124

Kerns, R., 107

Kessler, R., 34

Kewman, D., 151

King, S., 128

Kissane, D., 137

Kleepsies, P., 145

knee problems, 118, 160

Kopp, M., 108

Koskela, K., 48

Kriegsman, D., 132–3

Kristjansdottir, G., 108, 144, 157

Kwentus, J., 126, 128

Kyle, D., 170

Kyriacou, D., 52

Laatsch, L., 8–9

Lafreniere, K., 43

Lalinec-Maced, M., 16, 18
Latina women's study, 66
Lawrence, D., 149
Lawton, M., 105, 128
Lazarsfeld, P., 45
legal circumstances, 144, 146, 157
LeGrand, J., 14
Leventhal, E.A., 67
Lewis, G., 143
Liang, M., 128
libido, 103, 104, 107, 189
Lieberman, M., 133
Liefbroer, A., 130
life stage, of family, 89, 90, 101
life-skills development, 84, 86, 93,
    100
limb, loss of, 3, 6ff. See also amputa-
    tion
Lobo, L., 53
loneliness, 130, 140, 144. See also
    alienation; isolation
long-term disability (LTD), 35, 54–6
loss: categories of losses, 188;
    definition of, 22; restoration of,
    190–1; and reversals, 97–8. See
    under specific losses mentioned
loss of roles. See roles
loss of self-esteem. See self-esteem
loss-orientation, 167, 174, 183, 191
Lower, N., 9
lupus, 125, 129
Lynch, M., 146, 164

Maciejewski, P., 34
Maes, M., 105
Mahiacek, M., 137
malingering, 69

Malkinson, R., 137
Mantyselka, P., 30
Marino, J., 16
marital conflict, 17, 19, 25, 30, 31, 32,
    34, 52, 54, 76, 87, 105, 123, 130,
    156, 158
Marotz-Baden, R., 53
marriage, and roles in, 29–31, 36, 37,
    38, 53, 57–9, 66, 67, 73, 75, 81, 85,
    92, 94, 96, 103, 117, 119, 121, 122,
    124, 129, 131, 139, 146, 158, 159,
    161, 173, 174, 177, 178, 180
marriage therapy, 95, 158–9
Maruta, T., 111
Matthews, K., 105
Mayer, M., 132
McCaffery, M., 150–1
McCamish-Svensson, C., 130
McDonald, K., 70
McGaughey, D., 70
McGuigan, J., 107
McMaster Model Family Function-
    ing, 84, 96–8
meaning, and meaning-making, 45,
    61, 66, 80, 93, 99, 100, 102, 165,
    175, 176
medical condition, 26, 37, 41, 45, 75,
    101, 113, 119, 163, 166, 168, 184
medical-social perspective, 155
melanoma, 93
Melanson, P., 128
Melding, P., 128
Melzack, R., 127
memory loss, 125, 131
men, and masculinity, 69, 75, 78, 80,
    89, 104, 105, 109, 117, 118, 130,
    154, 156, 157, 164, 177

menopause, 20, 106
menses, 177
mental health, 105, 149, 152, 187
mental illness, 19, 30, 51, 145, 147, 149
metastasis, 147
Meunier, G., 131
mid-life, 105, 111
migraine, 28, 79, 84, 85. *See also* headache
Miller, E., 22
Mishra, S., 130
mismanagement of pain, 127
Monahan, D., 130
Monga, T., 111
Montenero, P., 111
mood, 59, 105, 162, 172; disorder, 38, 40, 41, 60
Moss, M., 105, 128
mother, and mothering, 3–4, 69, 83, 85, 88–90, 98, 105, 106, 114, 116, 126, 134, 139, 160, 176, 179, 180, 182
motivation, patient's, 77, 169
motor vehicle accident. *See* automobile accident
mourning, 3, 5, 14, 16, 17, 19, 21, 42, 61, 65, 115, 140, 165, 168; conditions affecting the course of, 27
multiple sclerosis, 26, 62, 170
musculoskeletal pain, 128
mutilation, 6
myocardial infarction, 94
myofascial pain syndrome, 93

narcotic analgesic, 72, 155
Nathawat, S., 10

Nau, D., 171
neck pain, 35, 39–40
Neimeyere, R., 137, 167–8
neurological degenerative symptoms, 128
neurological investigations, 160
Newman, A., 109
Niskanen, L., 48
Nord, D., 70
Norwegian studies, 47–8
numbness, 5, 136
nursing home, 129, 131, 133, 138; studies, 128

Omarzu, J., 22
Orbell, S., 50
Oriol, W., 127
orthopaedic investigations, 160
Osborne, D., 111
Osterweil, D., 128
outcome, 24, 27, 34–5, 81; studies, 137, 168–70, 185

pain assessment 127
pain clinic, 32, 35, 40, 44, 170, 172, 174, 178, 181
pain in old age, 126ff
pain management, 125, 141
Pain Research and Management, 126
pain-depression relationship, 22, 27, 109, 170
Papagiannidou, S., 13
parent, parenting, 7, 13, 18, 36, 62, 63, 73, 75, 76, 81, 83, 91, 108, 113, 114, 120, 158, 173, 180, 181
Parera, N., 145

Parkes, M., 4–10, 14, 19–25, 30–4, 136, 140, 169
Parkinson's disease, 26
Parmalee, P., 128
partner, loss of, 7, 25, 29–35
partner abuse, 52
partner relationship, 68. *See also* marriage
passive-aggressive behaviour, 85
pediatrician, 115
peers, 113, 115, 182, 185
pelvic pain, 17, 116
Penkower, L., 53
Penninx, B., 132–3
Peregoy, J., 53
persistent pain, 186. *See also* chronic pain
personality changes, 57, 59. *See also* identity
Peters, A., 130
Peterson, Y., 111
phantom limb, 6
phase-task approach, 184, 187
physical capacity, 63
physical condition, 113, 133
physical functions, loss of, 8, 64, 173
physical therapy, 169
Poli, P. 146
Poole, J., 83
post-menopausal women, 20
post-traumatic stress disorder (PTSD), 8
Potashnik, S., 133
poverty, 8, 38, 40, 46, 51, 97. *See also* financial circumstances
predictability, 172. *See also* unpredictability

pregnancy, 35, 151
Price, D., 126
Prigerson, H., 34
prostate conditions, 103, 109
prosthetics, 9, 10, 169, 189
prostitution, 117
Pruchno, R., 133
psychiatric assessment, 41, 110, 127
psychiatric consequences of loss, 9, 11, 15, 81, 93, 112–13, 135
psychiatric disorders, and chronic pain, 21, 40, 47, 107, 147, 190
psychiatry, 40
psychoanalytic approaches, 168, 171
psychological distress, 9, 10, 14, 23, 43, 60, 63, 66, 72, 76, 81, 83, 84, 92, 98, 102, 107, 108, 109, 132, 135, 146, 151, 153, 155, 162, 163, 173, 191
psychologist, 152
psychosocial assessment, 20, 57, 91, 164
psychosocial factors, 6, 20, 26, 107, 109, 111, 113
psychotherapeutic intervention. *See* psychotherapy
psychotherapy, 28, 39, 58, 63, 64, 65, 76, 77, 138, 141, 155, 165, 167, 169, 170, 172, 174
psychotropic drugs, 171
Puig, C., 145

radiological investigations, 160
Randolph, J., 27
randomized controlled trials, 109. *See also* outcome studies
rape, 188

Raphael, B., 12
Rau, M., 171
recognition, 165
recovery, 13–14, 24, 66, 70, 76, 80–1, 90
Reed, L., 28, 137
rehabilitation, 9, 12, 169, 172, 190
'reinvent' oneself, 170, 175. *See also* identity
Reisine, S., 83
rejection, feelings of, 123
religion, 113
relocation (of home), 3, 7, 8
reproductive capacity, 12. *See also* fertility
resentment, 29, 38, 96, 100
residual abilities, 166; assessment of, 191
resiliency, human, 62, 163, 176, 181, 183
resolution, 168, 184
restoration phase, 167, 175, 179, 180
restoration-orientation, 167, 191
Rethelyi, J., 108
retirement, 78, 91, 94, 95, 140
retraining, 187
Revenson, T., 83
rheumatoid arthritis, 22, 39–40, 74, 75, 76, 81, 109, 110, 128, 150, 172–3, 175, 184; and grief therapy, 172–6; and loss of roles, 56–8, 63–8, 83; and suicide, 150
Rhodes, V., 46
rib pain, 129
robbery, 188
Roeske, N., 14

roles, loss of, 26, 38, 39, 45, 56–8, 63–8, 75–7, 83–102, 125–6, 130–1, 134, 138, 153, 156–7, 166, 170, 171–6, 179, 180, 184, 187–8, 190–1; and grief therapy, 45–7. *See also* chronic sick role; employment; family roles; job loss
Rooparinesingh, S., 14
Rose, M., 112
Rosenheck, R., 34
Rowe, J., 128
Roy, R., 24, 45–6, 50, 75, 83–4, 88–90, 111, 124, 127–8
Royall, D., 106
Rubin, A., 111
Rubin, S., 135
Rumzek, H., 43
Ruskin, O., 131

sadness, 27, 28, 29, 32–4, 37–8, 42, 55, 80, 96, 99, 101, 102, 107, 115, 120, 122, 174, 187
safe sex, 70
scarring, 113
Schechter, N., 135
Schliebner, C., 53
Schoffling, K., 111
Scholz, O., 111
school, 30, 36, 40, 73, 87, 91, 113, 114, 117, 161, 162, 163, 181
Schulz, R., 132
Schut, H., 137, 167
Scott, B., 132
seizure, 145
self-definition, 62, 67–8, 72, 78. *See also* identity

self-esteem, 18, 37, 39, 44, 46–50, 65, 66, 77, 80, 108, 144, 157, 163, 166, 175, 176, 188
self-identity. *See* identity
self-recrimination, 117
Sengstaken, E., 128
separation, marital, 36–7
sexual function, 12–14, 16, 18, 38, 103–6, 109–13, 118–20, 122–3, 154, 174
Shahani, B., 8–9
shame, 39, 47, 69, 88, 109, 117–18, 136, 190
Shanas, E., 131
Shanks-McElroy, H., 132
Shapiro, E., 137
Sheeran, P., 50
shock, 29, 47, 109, 136
shoulder pain, 160
Siddique, C., 43
Silver, R., 33
single parent, 69
sleep disturbance, 6, 136, 162
social factors and roles, 10, 17, 40, 44, 47, 50, 60, 73, 74, 81, 82, 102, 109, 110, 113, 117, 124, 127, 136, 139, 141, 146, 148, 150–1, 153, 177, 187, 191
social support, 24, 30–1, 66, 70, 80–1, 114, 131–4, 134, 138–9, 145, 182
society, 20, 68, 69, 75, 190
somatization, 24, 27, 33, 34, 106, 107, 108, 138–40, 144, 155
somatization disorder, 107
spinal cord injury, 151–2
spinal stenosis, 125

spousal relationship, 103, 122. *See also* marriage
spouse, loss of, 3
Stang, P., 43
Starkey, J., 53–4
Steiner, M., 14
Sternbach, R., 128
stigma, 45, 69, 70, 72, 127
Stoller, E., 127
stomach pain. *See* abdominal pain
stress, 10, 31, 76–7, 85, 88, 98, 131–4, 144, 157; and unemployment, 44, 49, 53–4
Strobino, J., 132
Stroebe, M., 137, 167
Stroebe, W., 167
stroke, 25–7
Structured Clinical Interview, 146–7
substance abuse, 151, 152, 168
suicide, 25, 40, 44, 47, 73, 77, 81, 143, 144, 156, 162, 168; and cancer, 145–50; and loss of identity, 153, 157; and pain, 150–3; reasons for, 142, 163–4
surgery, 9, 10, 11, 13, 14, 15, 17, 18, 19, 73, 113, 114, 115, 118, 120, 182
Suris, J., 145
Sveinbjarnardottir, E., 108, 144, 157
Swami, D., 10
Swedish studies, 48–9, 130, 148, 150
Swensen, C., 171
symbolic bond or meaning, 11, 44, 58, 168. *See also* meaning (psychological)
symptomatic consequences, of losses, 168

tachycardia, 91
Takala, E., 108
Tan, G., 111–12
Tate, D., 151
Tebb, S., 132
teenager, 113, 115, 123, 145, 172, 182
terminally ill patient, 143
Tewksbury, R., 70
theory of grief, 7, 22, 32, 188
theory of loss, 3
therapeutic intervention, 137. *See also various therapies and treatments*
Thomas, K., 128
Thomas, M., 24, 88, 90, 126–8
Thompson, S., 22, 170
tranquilllizer, 154, 155
transference, 168
trauma, 30, 41, 42, 44–5, 98, 103, 122, 133–4, 168, 171, 189; wartime, 8
treatment plan, 166. *See also various therapies*
Tunks, E., 83
Turk, D., 111
Turpin, T., 16

uncertainty, 173, 185
unemployment, 45, 60–1; depression and, 43, 48–9, 51, 58–9, 61; and family, 50–4, 56; and grief, 26, 44, 46; stress and, 44, 53–4; and suicide, 44, 47. *See also* employment; job loss; work
unpredictability, of course of losses, 22, 41–2, 65–6, 70, 184, 185. *See also* predictability
urinary urgency, 112

uterus, loss of, 14, 182

vaginoplasty, 113, 181
Vali, F., 27
Valkenberg, H., 128
van Eijk, T., 132–3
Vanger, P., 110
vascular diseases, 128
Verkasalo, M., 108
Verma, S., 27
Veum, J., 50
victimization, 190
Viinamaeki, H., 48
Vilhjalmsson, R., 108, 144, 157
Vinokur, A., 44
violence, 44, 51–4, 59–60, 116–18, 121, 126
Vitaliano, P., 132
volunteer/volunteering, 64, 77, 130, 175
von Korff, M., 43

Wade, T., 53
Walkup, J., 27
Watkins, G., 53
Webb, A., 53
weight loss, 6, 162
Weiss, R., 22–5, 30, 34, 140, 188
welfare, social, 156
West Indian women's study, 14
white-collar workers, 43, 44, 53, 54
Whitley-Reed, L., 83, 170
widow/er, 6, 23, 25, 30, 31, 33, 129
wife, and role of, 5, 54, 59, 73, 76, 78, 80, 90, 92, 95, 96, 97, 98, 100, 102, 132, 152, 154, 157, 159, 173, 174, 176, 179

Williams, A., 26–7
Williamson, G., 9
Wink, P., 106
Winokuer, H., 140
Witte, E., 53
women, and femininity, 8, 10, 13, 14, 16–18, 20, 49, 69, 71, 89, 133, 142, 150–1, 174, 180, 181, 183, 185, 188
work, 28, 31, 38; meaning of, 44, 68; role of, 26, 43–4, 47, 52–3, 56–7, 68–9, 83, 98, 172–3, 187–9, 190. *See also* employment; job loss

work-site accident, 38
workers' compensation, 38, 46, 153–6
Wortman, C., 33–4

Xu, H., 144

Yee, J., 132

Zakham, L., 16
Zautra, A., 24
Zeisel, H., 45